Clinical Supervision for Nurses

Clinical Supervision for Nurses

Lisa Lynch
Kerrie Hancox
Brenda Happell

and

Judith Parker

WILEY-BLACKWELL

A John Wiley & Sons, Ltd., Publication

Blackwell Publishing was acquired by John Wiley & Sons in February 2007.
Blackwell's publishing programme has been merged with Wiley's global
Scientific, Technical, and Medical business to form Wiley-Blackwell.

Registered office
John Wiley & Sons Ltd, The Atrium, Southern Gate, Chichester, West Sussex,
PO19 8SQ, United Kingdom

Editorial office
9600 Garsington Road, Oxford, OX4 2DQ, United Kingdom
350 Main Street, Malden, MA 02148-5020, USA

For details of our global editorial offices, for customer services and for
information about how to apply for permission to reuse the copyright
material in this book please see our website at
www.wiley.com/wiley-blackwell.

Library of Congress Cataloging-in-Publication Data

Clinical supervision for nurses / Lisa Lynch . . . [et al.].
p. ; cm.
Includes bibliographical references and index.
ISBN 978-1-4051-6059-9 (pbk. : alk. paper)   1. Nurses–Supervision of.
I. Lynch, Lisa, 1973–
[DNLM: 1. Nursing Care–organization & administration.   2. Nursing,
Supervisory.   3. Clinical Competence.   4. Clinical Medicine–organization &
administration. WY 105 C6408 2008]
RT86.45.C55 2008
610.73–dc22
2008013046

A catalogue record for this book is available from the British Library.

Set in 10 on 12 pt Palatino by SNP Best-set Typesetter Ltd., Hong Kong
Printed in Singapore by C.O.S. Printers Pte Ltd

1   2008

Contents

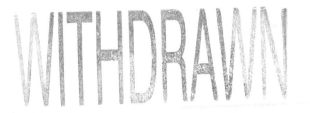

About the authors

Lisa Lynch
Southern Health
Lisa Lynch is the Director of Child and Adolescent Mental Health and Primary Partnerships at Southern Health and the Co-Director of Clinical Supervision Consultants. She has been involved with clinical supervision, as a supervisor, a supervisee, a manager and an academic, for more than 10 years. She is a passionate advocate for nurses receiving access to appropriate clinical supervision. Lisa was a co-developer of the fully accredited *Clinical Supervision for Health Care Professionals* course, and the workshop for potential supervisees *Unlocking the Secret,* both introduced in Victoria in 2001. These highly successful programs were amongst the first of their kind. Lisa has recently completed a Master of Nursing by Research. Lisa undertook a study of the implementation of clinical supervision in a mental health service in Victoria. The findings from her work culminated in a model to guide the implementation of clinical supervision within health care settings, now known as the Lynch model.

Kerrie Hancox
Southern Health
Kerrie Hancox is Co-Director of Clinical Supervision Consultants. She also works in primary mental health and in enhanced crisis and assessment. She has been working in psychiatry since 1985 in a wide variety of clinical settings in Australia and overseas. Kerrie has a Bachelor of Nursing and completed her Master in Psychiatric Nursing in 2000. The focus of her research was clinical supervision. Kerrie has skills and expertise in a range of therapeutic skills, including family therapy and gestalt therapy. She also has expertise in organisational dynamics and socio analysis education. Kerrie is currently a board member of the

Australian College of Mental Health Nurses. Kerrie was co-developer with Lisa Lynch of *Clinical Supervision for Health Care Professionals* and *Unlocking the Secret*. She remains committed to the importance of quality education for supervisors and supervisees.

Brenda Happell
Central Queensland University

Brenda is the Professor of Contemporary Nursing at Central Queensland University. In her former position as the inaugural Director of the Centre for Psychiatric Nursing Research and Practice, Brenda was responsible for identifying the need for, and subsequently overseeing the development of, the subject *Clinical Supervision for Health Care Professionals* and she is currently a member of the Clinical Supervision Taskforce for Queensland Health. Brenda is nationally and internationally recognised for her expertise in nursing, as evidenced by invitations as a visiting scholar and to present at national and international conferences. Brenda has published prolifically in nursing and related health journals and her work is frequently cited and used to effect practice change. Brenda is currently the Editor of the *International Journal of Mental Health Nursing* and Associate Editor of *Issues in Mental Health Nursing*. Brenda is an Honorary Professor at the University of Alberta and the University of Texas (Tyler).

Judith Parker
Victoria University

Professor Judith Parker AM has played a major role in the development of nursing programs and research in the university sector in Australia. She was the foundation Professor and Head of the School of Nursing at the University of Melbourne from 1996 to March 2004. Prior to that, she was foundation Professor and Head of the School of Nursing at La Trobe University. Professor Parker initiated the establishment of two centres for nursing research at the University of Melbourne, both of which are dedicated to conducting research leading to the improvement of clinical nursing practice. Under Professor Parker's leadership the School of Nursing obtained a large number of research grants, several of which Professor Parker has been actively involved in. Professor Parker is internationally renowned for her research into the nursing handover, which was funded by the Australian Research Council (ARC) Large Grants Scheme. Her interest in clinical supervision builds upon the handover work. She is currently a principal investigator in the National Health and Medical Research Council funded Centre for Clinical Research Excellence in Neurosciences, 2003–8. Currently she is Head of the School of Nursing and Midwifery at Victoria University. Professor Parker established and was foundation Editor and later Editor in Chief of the very successful and highly regarded international refereed scholarly journal *Nursing Inquiry*, of which she is now Asia

Pacific Editor. In 2001 Professor Parker was included on the Victorian Honour Roll for Women and in 2002 she was made a Member of the General Division of the Order of Australia. In 2006 she was awarded an honorary Doctor of Medicine by the University of Melbourne in recognition of her contribution to nursing scholarship.

Foreword by Rosemary Bryant

This is an extremely timely publication. The shortage of nurses is a serious problem world wide and it is clear that not enough is being done to support and retain the nurses who are already working within the health care system. Clinical supervision can assist retention and this book makes a contribution to both clarifying the dimensions of clinical practice and offering sound practical advice on implementation and evaluation.

This book is the work of highly experienced professionals who have deep understanding of the issues that confront nurses in their daily practice. A particular strength of this book is that it focuses upon the importance of the local and particular contexts of practice and cautions against a 'one size fits all' approach to clinical supervision.

The authors clearly identify the hazards involved in implementing clinical supervision in an organisation. The book works well as a resource and practical guide for those wanting to introduce clinical supervision across an organisation and offers useful strategies that will assist in setting realistic processes and timeframes.

Currently there is considerable confusion about the meaning of the term 'clinical supervision'. This book clarifies many of the perplexing issues that surround the term and demonstrates the benefits of clinical supervision for nurses in a variety of practice settings. Although the book is designed for a nursing audience it would be a useful guide for other practice professionals. The book contains many scenarios of how clinical supervision works in practice. These are drawn from actual experience and highlight many of the interwoven ethical, legal, organisational and power issues that surround nursing practice which the process of clinical supervision seeks to unravel, clarify and provide guidance for.

Rosemary Bryant
Executive Director of Royal College of Nursing Australia
and
Second Vice President of the International Council of Nurses

Foreword by Peter Santangelo

Clinical supervision is not a new concept to nursing and its implementation in workplaces has been the aspiration of many a passionate and assertive nursing leader. Uptake, however, has been very slow, despite recognition that reflective practice is not only desirable, but a necessary facet of nursing professional development.

This publication offers comprehensive coverage of all the issues needing to be considered in relation to clinical supervision. It is a practical guide for implementation, with thoughtful deliberations on the underpinning principles of clinical supervision and sound methods by which it can be evaluated.

With vignettes and case studies strategically placed throughout the book, it makes its message very accessible to students, beginning and experienced practitioners, and to organisations who employ nurses to take charge of client care. The evidence base for its assertions are thorough, making it a truly authoritative resource that can provide the where-with-all to make clinical supervision achievable in all work settings.

The authors are to be congratulated for bringing all this together in one volume. The potential of this book for encouraging practice development and professional workplace health and safety is significant. It is hoped that these opportunities will be grasped by individual nurses and organisational managers alike.

Peter Santangelo
President, Australian College of Mental Health Nurses

Preface

The inspiration to write this book came, at least in part, from consideration of two important interrelated features of the nursing profession: the integral role nurses play in ensuring the safe and effective delivery of health care and the stress and burnout that nurses experience through their proximity to human distress. The continuing shortage of nurses can be in part explained by these factors and clinical supervision is put forward here as a structured means of assisting in the reduction of stress and burnout.

Nursing practice requires a strong educational base reflecting the acquisition of skills, knowledge and expertise necessary to meet contemporary health care challenges. Nurses are expected to advocate on behalf of their patients by challenging treatments when they believe the safety or well-being of patients is likely to be compromised. Nurses are continually encouraged to reflect on their practice and to consider how things could be done better or more effectively.

At the same time, the widely documented shortage of nurses not only continues but appears to be worsening. The inability to recruit sufficient nurses to meet health care needs is providing the impetus to introduce untrained and unregulated health workers to undertake some nursing roles. Understanding ways to retain nurses within the system is crucial for the viability of the nursing profession and to maintain quality within the health care system.

Our interest in these features lies in their implications for clinical supervision. Yes, nurses need to reflect on their practice but they need an accepted and acknowledged space to do this effectively. Reflective skills need to be valued within the health care system. Clinical supervision provides an ideal opportunity for nurses to reflect in a structured and purposeful way, with the assistance of a skilled person to work with individual nurses to help them to meet pre-determined goals.

Nursing is a stressful profession and burnout is not an uncommon experience. The stress associated with nursing has repeatedly been identified as a reason why many nurses leave their chosen profession and seek employment in a non-health related field. There is some evidence to suggest that clinical supervision can reduce stress levels and protect nurses from burnout. Clinical supervision should therefore be a crucial component of a successful recruitment strategy.

Writing this book reflects the authors' passion for and commitment to clinical supervision as central to nursing practice. It also acknowledges the fact that clinical supervision does not just happen because someone decides it is a good thing. It requires a structured process that is adapted to suit the prevailing culture of the specific organisation. The lack of a systematic implementation plan is one of the major reasons why clinical supervision does not succeed. A major strength of this book is the introduction of a model to guide the implementation process. The Lynch model was directly developed from practice and therefore reflects the issues, barriers and strategies associated with clinical supervision as experienced rather than from a purely theoretical perspective.

This is a very practical book. It deals with a range of issues from implementation through to clinical supervision in action. The book is set within a context of practice development. Approaches to and models of clinical supervision are discussed in detail to help potential supervisors to find a style that suits them. The clinical supervisory relationship is explored with handy hints for both supervisors and supervisees to secure the best fit between the two roles. Broader contextual issues such as law and ethics are examined specifically in relation to clinical supervision. Finally, evaluation is addressed as a way to determine the impact of clinical supervision and strengthen the case for its sustainability. The style of the book is engaging and conversational. Theoretical concepts are supported with scenarios, and a number of exercises have been included to encourage reflection. Models specifically developed by two of the authors have also been featured.

We hope you find the book a useful tool to support the implementation of clinical supervision in your organisation.

Good luck.

Acknowledgements

The authors would like to acknowledge:

- Alan Robins for expressing the initial interest in the education of clinical supervisors
- Linda Curtis and Anne Gumpold for their leadership in and facilitation of clinical supervision research
- Chris Pavlou for her supportive work in the area of clinical supervision
- Teresa Kelly for her expertise about the Peplau model
- the nurses and health care services who supported education as a necessary part of clinical supervision
- our partners, our children and our close friends. Writing a book is a time-consuming and absorbing process. Sometimes the greatest sacrifices are made by those close to the authors.

Particular thanks to Steve whose patience and support is never ending . . . the wind beneath my wings. (BH)

An introduction to clinical supervision

Introduction

The primary aims of this chapter are to:

- provide an overview of the intention, structure and format of this book
- consider the benefits of clinical supervision for nurses
- examine and refute common myths and misconceptions about clinical supervision
- distinguish clinical supervision from other formal relationships, including managerial supervision, preceptorship, mentorship and therapy
- consider definitions of clinical supervision
- consider the development of clinical supervision within a wide range of nursing specialties.

About this book

The aim of this book is to provide an introduction as a guide to nurses with an interest in clinical supervision. It is intended that this book will assist the reader to:

- understand the meaning of clinical supervision and be able to clearly distinguish it from other forms of supervision
- appreciate the benefits of clinical supervision for practice development
- identify the complexity of clinical supervision from both an individual and an organisational perspective

- recognise the roles and responsibilities that must be assumed by management, supervisors and supervisees if clinical supervision is to be successfully implemented
- utilise the book as a practical guide to assist with the implementation process
- assist with the development of the knowledge and skills required for the roles of supervisor and supervisee.

This book is presented in a user-friendly style to enhance its use as a practical resource guide. It is intended to be a useful guide for nurses, ranging from those with no prior knowledge to those who want to further enhance their knowledge and expand their skills as a supervisor, supervisee or both. A particular benefit of this book is that it emphasises and continually reminds us that we need to be familiar with the impact of the context in which clinical supervision will occur.

The book is also intended as a resource to guide the implementation of clinical supervision. It provides a step-by-step guide on how to implement clinical supervision and hence will be of considerable benefit to health care organisations, managers, senior nurses or clinicians seeking to introduce clinical supervision in their team, program or across an entire organisation. This book will help them to understand the implications and pitfalls, whilst also providing useful strategies that assist in setting realistic timelines and achievable goals.

Despite the increase in popularity of clinical supervision there is a paucity of literature, especially any pertaining to the implementation of clinical supervision or that considers implementation in an Australian context. The degree of success associated with the introduction of clinical supervision is likely to reflect preparation on a number of levels, including knowledge, organisational readiness, education and ongoing, demonstrable commitment. This Australian-based text presents an invaluable resource for managers, clinicians and educators alike.

This book is intended to be interactive rather than purely directive. You will be encouraged throughout to consider the topics and issues as they relate to what you hope to achieve from introducing clinical supervision in your organisation. To achieve this, a number of reflective exercises are included. Where possible, it is recommended that you complete these with the people who are likely to be part of, or important to, your implementation strategy.

Exercises and activities have also been developed to encourage reflection and skill development in the actual practice of clinical supervision, to enable nurses to fulfil the roles of supervisor and supervisee safely and effectively.

Clinical supervision – the new panacea?

The recent surge in the popularity of clinical supervision for nursing might lead one to conclude that this is a new phenomenon, developed as a strategy to address the challenges, stresses and opportunities facing the nursing profession in the 21st century. On the contrary, in 1925 a clinical supervision conference was held at the annual Institute of New York State League of Nurse Education. The conference attracted 367 nurses from 61 hospitals '. . . an event that surely reflected the level of interest shown in supervision at a time ready for changes in nursing practice' (Yegdich, 1999: 1196).

These words could be uttered today and lose none of their relevance. The need and opportunity for nursing practice to develop and respond to changes in health care needs and the structure of the health care system remains an issue of pressing concern. Given the importance attributed to clinical supervision so long ago, why is it not already an inherent part of contemporary nursing practice? Why do we appear to have made so little advancement with an initiative that should be central to contemporary nursing practice?

Why do we need clinical supervision?

If I cannot help me I cannot help you

Many of us have travelled by air on at least one occasion and are likely to have heard the routine safety instructions at the beginning of the flight. As part of this we are instructed how to secure the oxygen mask and advised to secure our own mask before assisting others such as children. While the rationale for this is not explicitly stated, it is probably obvious to most, especially to nurses, who know that without sufficient oxygen flow our cognitive function is likely to be impaired and our capacity to assist others will be seriously compromised. Such a statement is necessary because of the natural tendency most of us have to put the health and safety of others, particularly those who depend on us, above our own well-being.

This example serves as a particularly apt analogy to introduce the importance of clinical supervision for nursing. In order to provide the highest level of support and expertise to those we care for professionally, we must ensure that we are in the best possible shape to do so; in short we must look after ourselves.

A fundamental aim of this book is to articulate the important role of clinical supervision in assisting nurses to look after themselves professionally in order to provide the highest possible standard of care.

Clinical supervision is sometimes criticised for being about nurses rather than patients. It may be considered as a self-indulgent or feel-good activity that detracts from nurses focusing on the real purpose of their work. Such a view appears to assume that the interests of nurses and patients are mutually exclusive. We do not support this view – you cannot adequately care for one without the other. It is, of course, extremely important that patient care is as good as it can be. However, this will only occur if we value the well-being of the people delivering the care. Clinical supervision is a valid process for the well-being of nurses as individuals and as health professionals.

Nurses are human

Many of us undertook our nursing education or training within a culture that espoused the importance of detachment. 'Don't get emotionally involved' was a common phrase, based on the assumption that nurses needed some degree of distance from their patients to ensure they would provide effective care; too much emotion was considered unprofessional. This also reflected the view that nurses must switch off from their own personal views and opinions in order to ensure a non-judgemental approach to care. In short, nurses were encouraged to become mechanical providers of care and shelve their personality and humanity for the duration of the shift.

Clinical supervision is therefore an important part of ensuring that nurses look after themselves and face their own views and prejudices in order to work effectively with a broad array of stakeholders within the health care environment, including nurses, other health care professionals, patients and their families and significant others. Effective clinical supervision acknowledges the 'humanness' of nurses. It can teach us how to use our personalities, skills and knowledge to form positive and constructive relationships and interactions. Clinical supervision can also help us identify the aspects of our behaviour that might get in the way of our interactions and relationships. We do not wake up in the morning and put on our nurse outfit and head off to work. We are not mechanical providers of health care – we continue to be people with views, prejudices and judgements throughout the working day.

Remember we all:

- have our own beliefs/value system
- have good and bad days
- have things that 'push our buttons' or annoy us
- use ourselves as a 'tool' in the work that we do with our patients.

Clinical supervision – more than making us feel good

While caring for the carer is important, clinical supervision encompasses the development and improvement of the nurse's practice as an individual and as part of a team. As professionals most of us would agree that learning and development occur throughout our careers and that even the most experienced nurse has a great deal to learn. Clinical supervision provides a framework to facilitate life-long learning and to enable the nurse to develop the knowledge and skills he or she requires to practice within a dynamic health care environment.

But I do not have time for clinical supervision

Most of you are probably thinking there are not enough hours in the day already to do what needs to be done, let alone find time to attend clinical supervision sessions. Clinical supervision needs to become a valued part of practice that is considered an essential aspect of a nurse's role, just like the clinical handover. Participating in handover is not an option, it is not something we do if we can find the time; it is an essential part of the role of a nurse and seen as an important tool in providing good clinical care to patients. Unfortunately, many nurses do not make time for clinical supervision or if they do it may be the first thing they drop to attend to other demands when work gets particularly busy. Valuing clinical supervision as a non-negotiable part of a nurse's role is essential if it is to become as embedded a part of professional practice as other nursing obligations such as the handover.

Example

Take the example of the woodchopper who is given a short length of time to chop a field of trees. He doesn't stop for a break, just flies into the task. A passer-by notices that the axe the woodchopper is using is a little blunt and asks him why he doesn't stop to sharpen the axe. The woodchopper replies that he does not have time to stop and sharpen the axe; he just has to keep on chopping as he has to chop all the trees in the area before the end of the day. The passer-by keeps walking and the woodchopper just keeps on chopping.

The passer-by knows, as we do, that if the woodchopper stopped to sharpen his axe he would get the job done more effectively and efficiently. However, as the woodchopper feels the pressure to keep going, it is possible the job will not be done by the deadline.

This analogy is easily applied to a day in the life of a nurse. On a daily basis there are many tasks to complete by the end of the shift and enormous pressure to get them all done. Often there does not appear to be enough time to stop, to reflect, to slow down and check to see if everything is working properly or see if things could be done differently and more efficiently.

While we are busy doing things we do not allow ourselves the space to think about how we can do them differently and perhaps even more efficiently or effectively. The risk is that our practice becomes robotic and static; we do not take the time to consider different ways of doing things or keeping pace with the latest trends. Increasingly, we tend to feel as though we are responding to immediate demands rather than making a real difference, we can become dissatisfied with our role and cease to practice as effectively as we used to.

Consider clinical supervision as an investment: the time spent on it produces results that far outweigh the time it takes.

Myths and confusion about clinical supervision

A clear understanding of what clinical supervision means continues to be elusive. A review of the literature on this topic since 1925 presents a wide variety of definitions. This absence of a universally accepted definition has resulted in many misunderstandings or myths associated with clinical supervision. Indeed, the actual term 'clinical supervision' is a likely contributor to these myths.

Taken literally the term 'supervision' means overseeing or having vision over. Clinical supervision therefore literally means overseeing someone's clinical practice. To many nurses this equates to a 'nurse supervisor' role that directs, inspects and controls nurses' clinical work. It is therefore considered by many nurses to be a form of surveillance where the supervised nurse is observed to ensure his or her practice is of an acceptable standard and held accountable if it fails to do so.

There are many examples in the literature, particularly from the UK in the 1990s, that have contributed to confusion for nurses between clinical 'snoopervision' and clinical supervision. During this time clinical supervision was seen as an essential part of clinical governance and phrases such as 'protection of clients' (Simms, 1993: 329) 'fundamental to safe guarding standards' and 'the major force in improving clinical standards and enhancing the quality of care' (Moores, 1994: 3) procured a sense of surveillance. Nurses tend to think of words such as quality, governance, safety, protection, and monitoring as the function of managers, not clinical supervisors (Consedine, 1994). As a result of this confusion and the absence of a broadly accepted definition, a number of myths and misconceptions have developed about clinical supervision.

An article by Mackereth (1996) suggested that for clinical supervision to be welcomed and effective it must be viewed as useful, safe and appropriate to the supervisee's practice. He also identified eight misconceptions about clinical supervision that present significant barriers to clinical supervision being viewed as positive. These misconceptions have been noted in other clinical supervision literature and are often identified as one of the reasons clinical supervision is not universally accepted by nurses and implemented throughout organisations. In the authors' experience these misconceptions are expressed by nurses again and again, whenever clinical supervision is discussed. In a series of workshops conducted by two of the authors, discussing and then dispelling these myths has been necessary before being able to move onto more general discussions about clinical supervision. The eight misconceptions identified by Mackereth (1996: 39) have included supervision being seen as:

(1) an informal and ad hoc arrangement or interaction
(2) a dumping ground or whinge session
(3) therapy for the supervisee or supervisor
(4) counselling or an opportunity to practice as a counsellor
(5) an opportunity to discipline, identify and eject 'bad' or 'unsuitable' nurses
(6) an imposed non-negotiable 'supervisory' arrangement controlled and delivered by managers
(7) an opportunity for senior nurses to be intimate with junior colleagues
(8) the supervisor having total accountability and responsibility for the supervisee's work.

You may have already encountered some of the above misconceptions and it is likely you will continue to do so in the future. In fact, some of you may have been thinking that one or more of these misconceptions were actually true. They are common thoughts about supervision and it is important that we now spend some time in this text dispelling these before we can move on.

(1) An informal and ad hoc arrangement or interaction

Nurses sometimes assume that clinical supervision is the same as the informal and ad hoc arrangements that they have created for themselves. When you ask nurses if they receive clinical supervision some nurses will say yes; however, many times they are actually referring to ad hoc arrangements: the brief catch ups in the medication or treatment room, discussions over morning tea or those 5-minute coffee breaks, the car rides on the way to community assessments or, in some cases, interactions at the pub after work. These are the times when we 'off load' or 'let off steam' to trusted colleagues. It might also be a time when we seek support or advice in working with a patient or group of patients we find particularly difficult or challenging, or spend time debriefing about a particularly difficult or sad event. In the absence of a formal structure for clinical supervision, many nurses will seek support through these informal processes.

This informal collegial support has very different structures, functions and meanings from clinical supervision. For example, clinical supervision is formal and structured. It occurs on a regular basis (for example weekly, fortnightly or monthly). Each session follows a structured format around aims, content and expectations, whereas our informal support networks really are informal ad hoc, spontaneous interactions. These informal supports serve a very important function and will never be replaced by the introduction of clinical supervision.

(2) A dumping ground or whinge session
Clinical supervision may be seen by some nurses as an opportunity to unload by complaining about colleagues, management or patients. Nurses may think that they can spend time in clinical supervision 'dumping' all of their issues and problems onto the supervisor. The intent of clinical supervision is far broader than this.

If concerns/complaints and issues are raised in supervision they should be discussed only in so far as they impact on professional practice. As clinical supervision is a formal and structured relationship, there needs to be a purpose to, and expectation of, an ultimate outcome from this exploration. If supervisees choose to talk about conflict or difficulties with other staff members, then the role they play in contributing to the conflict must be acknowledged and ways that the conflict or difficulty could be resolved must be identified and addressed.

In a clinical supervision session concerns or grievances may be explored, but the clinical supervisor should not collude by making statements like 'I know what you mean, people like that are hard work'. Rather, the supervisor should encourage the supervisee to identify his or her role within the conflict and explore ways that the conflict or difficulty could be resolved.

Example
Jane starts today's supervision session discussing a disagreement she had with a peer in the previous week. Jane begins by describing the incident but very quickly moves into listing all the things she dislikes about this nurse. In addition Jane states that everyone in the team feels the same way about this staff member and claims that nobody wants to work with her. When Jane is describing the incident she places blame 100% on the other nurse and reflects only on all the things the other nurse could have done to 'fix' the situation.

The supervisor's role in this example is not to agree with Jane, nor is it to allow Jane just to whinge and vent about the incident in a one-sided way. The role of the clinical supervisor is to assist Jane to reflect on the disagreement and her overall relationship with her peer in a more constructive and holistic way.

(3) Therapy for the supervisee or supervisor
and

(4) Counselling or an opportunity to practice as a counsellor
It is in fact a common misconception that clinical supervision is therapy for nurses, or even an opportunity for supervisors to practice their counselling skills. There are in fact many plausible reasons for why nurses think clinical supervision is therapy or practice for a trainee therapist. These include the history of supervision having a strong foundation in therapy and counselling, and the use of clinical supervision as a tool for training psychoanalysts and psychotherapists. In addition, many of the interpersonal skills and attributes of a clinical supervisor are essentially the same as good counselling skills or the characteristics of a counsellor. The lack of a clear definition that articulates the differences between therapy and supervision is also another contributing factor.

The process of clinical supervision itself has also been articulated as one of the reasons clinical supervision can be seen as therapy. It is a formal relationship and agreement between two people, there are regular sessions, usually for an hour in length, and the sessions take place in an office (generally that of the supervisor). If clinical supervision is provided privately a fee is paid for the service. This resembles the environment for therapy or a counselling session and this can sometimes be intimidating or scary for nurses who fear that clinical supervision is really therapy.

The purpose and function of supervision can also be seen as therapeutic and some nurses have even described supervision as 'work therapy'. While clinical supervision may make nurses feel more comfortable about their practice, the fundamental difference is that the focus is always a work context not a personal one.

Example

Mary is a 38-year-old woman who is desperately seeking to have a baby. After trying to conceive naturally for many years she has been undergoing IVF treatments for the past 2 years, but has not been able to become pregnant to date. Mary is working in a private maternity and gynaecology hospital. She is currently providing care for Jennifer, who has had five surgical terminations of pregnancy (STOP) during the past 15 months. Mary is finding it difficult to develop a caring relationship for Jennifer and other patients with a similar history.

At the suggestion of a colleague, Mary seeks clinical supervision. She describes her reaction to Jennifer and begins to talk about how unfair it is that while she cannot conceive, other women are 'throwing babies away'.

Reflective exercise

- What signs might warn you that Mary is moving from the professional to the personal domain?
- How would you as a supervisor assist Mary to focus on her professional practice rather than personal issues?

Possible signs that Mary may be moving from the professional into the personal:

- Avoidance of working with women in Jennifer's situation.
- Strong emotional responses when working with Jennifer, for example anger and impatience when Jennifer takes 'too long' to get out of bed.
- Giving Jennifer less time and care than she gives other patients.

An aim of clinical supervision is to increase supervisees' awareness of their own personal issues and how these might impact in the work environment.

The actions of Mary's clinical supervisor could be as follows:

- Assist Mary to talk about the quality of her relationship with Jennifer by considering how she interacts with her. Allow her time to talk about her experience of caring for Jennifer and other women who have had STOPs. What are the possible reasons Mary identifies that are getting in the way of her being able to form a caring relationship with Jennifer and those women in similar situations?
- The supervisor might also ask Mary about a patient that she really likes and ask her to imagine that she is interacting with her in the way she does with Jennifer. How would that feel? How is it different from how she is interacting with Jennifer? How would the patient be likely to react?
- Mary may need time to work through her feelings about nursing patients in Jennifer's situation – given that she works in a maternity and gynaecology hospital she is likely to come in contact with other patients in similar positions and Mary can use her clinical supervision to explore her past responses and future reactions.
- The supervisor may even guide Mary to reflect on her responses to patients who have had STOPs more than a year ago, prior to her having fertility problems. Were her responses different, was her experience of caring for these patients different? If so how?
- Depending on the level of Mary's distress and the impact these situations are having on her personally she may want to discuss the personal impact this is having on her with a fertility or IVF counsellor.

As her clinical supervisor it is not your role to provide therapy for Mary in relation to her infertility, it is your role to assist Mary to reflect on and explore the impact this personal experience has in relation to her work. In Mary's particular situation this means working with patients whom she perceives are 'throwing their babies away'.

(5) An opportunity to discipline, identify and eject 'bad' or 'unsuitable' nurses

The lines between clinical supervision and therapy, management and education are often seen as blurry and confusing. In the previous misconception we explored the lines between supervision and therapy, and in the final four misconceptions the differences between clinical supervision and education and management need to be clearly articulated.

There are concerns from a number of nurses that the goal or mission of a clinical supervisor is to utilise supervision sessions to identify and ultimately discipline and eject 'bad' or 'unsuitable' nurses. In reality some supervisors may be instructed by managers within the organisation to go on a 'seek and destroy' mission and hunt down all the 'bad' nurses and get rid of them. This is certainly not clinical supervision. Clinical supervision is a tool to support staff with strengths or limitations that they have themselves identified with the intention of encouraging nurses to acknowledge their limitations and feel sufficiently safe and secure to work towards overcoming them. This is not to suggest that 'seek and destroy' missions represent acceptable management practice either, but rather to emphasise that it is not within the ambit of clinical supervision to push this type of management agenda.

(6) An imposed non-negotiable 'supervisory' arrangement controlled and delivered by managers

It is a common misconception that clinical supervision is controlled by organisational management. It is often seen as synonymous or intertwined with line management. There is actually a logical reason for this common misconception. Currently, nursing registration bodies do not endorse clinical supervision or mandate it as a condition of registration (a practice which is common in other disciplines such as psychology). It is therefore the responsibility of individual organisations and hence management to 'allow' nurses access to clinical supervision. This means it is management who decide what clinical supervision is, who gets access to it, how it should be implemented or even whether or not they will support its implementation.

Although this means that line managers and organisations are involved in the overall implementation process, they have no role within the supervisory relationship itself. The content of supervision is between the clinical supervisor and clinical supervisee. The success of implementation of clinical supervision requires a clear delineation from line management. Table 1.1 demonstrates the essential difference between the two relationships.

Table 1.1   Line management vs clinical supervision.

	Line management	**Clinical supervision**
Definition	A hierarchical system of management structured like a pyramid, where authority and responsibility are passed downwards and accountability is passed upwards via line managers. http://www.allwords.com/word-line%20management.html	Clinical supervision is a formal process of consultation between two or more professionals. The focus is to provide support for the supervisee(s) in order to promote self-awareness, development and growth within the context of their professional environment (Hancox & Lynch, 2002: 6)
Participants	Paid employees from within the same organisation. Generally interviewed for the role. Line manager is appointed by the organisation. There is no choice of line manager.	Clinician–clinician, possibly from the same organisation but not necessarily. Generally, there should be some choice of supervisor and clinical supervision should always be voluntary.
Duration of relationship	For the length of the employment contract.	Ongoing, usually months or years for the length of the supervision agreement.
Frequency of contact	Often daily, formal and informal contact. Generally frequency of contact is determined by the line manager.	Defined in terms of relationship but commonly 1 hour per fortnight or as dictated by need between clinical supervisor and supervisee, that is at times the supervisee may request more or less frequent contact; this should always be negotiated and agreed to by both the supervisor and the supervisee.
Primary focus of relationship	To ensure staff members are fulfilling their role as employees, through the process of appraisal and ongoing monitoring and evaluation.	Multiple, includes organisational, professional and personal objectives.
Facilitator	Person who is appropriately experienced or trained in management.	An experienced, trained clinician 'supervisor', often from within supervisee's agency. Can be independent, external supervisor, of a number of disciplines.
Potential benefits	Support in the workplace, some capacity for learning and advancing skills through management functions such as succession planning and mentoring.	Learn, improve and refine clinical skills. Enhance reflective practice. Identify issues related to transference and counter-transference.

Continued

Table 1.1 *Continued*

	Line management	Clinical supervision
Limitations	Not all managers have the appropriate preparation for line management. They are accountable for their staff, therefore evaluators of their practice. It also may mean that they are involved in issues of performance management. This can obviously place strain on the relationship.	Availability of appropriately prepared clinical supervisors. Also the cost of training internal supervisors or providing access to private external supervisors can be prohibitive.
Aims of relationship	To ensure safe practice and the staff member working within organisational parameters to achieve key performance indicators.	Increase clinical/therapeutic skills. Provide support for clinicians within their professional life.

(7) An opportunity for senior nurses to be intimate with junior colleagues

Clinical supervision is not an opportunity for senior staff to spend time with their junior colleagues. Perhaps the development of this type of relationship could be thought of as a traditionally paternalistic one, or even a form of mentoring which provides an opportunity for the senior nurse to influence the junior nurse's growth and development in his or her own image. This is clearly not clinical supervision, which seeks to support nurses to develop their own potential.

(8) The supervisor having total accountability and responsibility for the supervisee's work

This is a misconception that frightens many budding supervisors as they feel an overwhelming sense of responsibility for the supervisee and fear that they will be held accountable for another nurse's practice. This is sometimes given as the reason nurses initially say no to the option of becoming a clinical supervisor. However, nurses are often confusing this with the registered nurse–student relationship, which is described in further detail below. Clinical supervision is a professional relationship between two qualified clinicians that is structured and formal, but accountability always remains with the supervisee. The supervisor provides the opportunity for the supervisee to explore approaches to his or her professional practice, but does not assume any responsibility for it. This concept will be explored in greater detail in the discussion of legal issues in Chapter 6.

Distinguishing clinical supervision from other relationships

In the above section, clinical supervision has been distinguished from therapy and line management. However, it is also commonly confused with preceptorship or mentorship. Table 1.2 provides an overview of the essential differences.

Reflective exercise

In addition to line management, therapy, preceptorship and mentorship there may be other forums in your organisation that either you or others around you have confused with clinical supervision.

Using Table 1.3 as a basis, list the similarities and differences between clinical supervision and these various other professional relationships that may be a feature of your organisational context.

You may do this individually but it would be more useful to complete the exercise as part of a group, preferably involving those people who are likely to be part of, or important to, your clinical supervision implementation strategy.

Reflective exercise

Are there any other professional forums or relationships in your organisation you think could be confused with clinical supervision? Using Table 1.4 add these other professional relationships, again exploring the similarities and differences between these relationships and clinical supervision.

Once you have completed this exercise refer to Table 1.5, which includes some ideas regarding the similarities and differences between clinical supervision and the forums and relationships covered above. This is certainly not intended as a complete or exhaustive list and we hope you have lots of additional ideas to add.

Towards a definition of clinical supervision

Distinguishing between clinical supervision and other relationships helps to provide clarity around the meaning of this term. However, given the confusion about what clinical supervision is and is not, the need for a clear definition is evident.

There is no one, universally agreed definition of clinical supervision. However, despite some differences between definitions there are many similarities. Most definitions include themes about professional

Table 1.2 Differentiating between preceptorship, mentorship and clinical supervision.

	Preceptorship	Clinical supervision	Mentorship
Definition	Preceptor – an experienced nurse who provides a supportive, educative one-to-one relationship to the preceptee/student.	Clinical supervision is a formal process of consultation between two or more professionals. The focus is to provide support for the supervisee(s) in order to promote self-awareness, development and growth within the context of their professional environment. (Hancox & Lynch, 2002).	Mentor – an experienced, trusted advisor or counsellor who offers helpful guidance to younger colleagues.
Participants	Student–clinician	Clinician–clinician	Clinician–clinician
Duration of relationship	Short term, often under 1 month.	Ongoing, usually months or years.	Ongoing, usually months or years.
Frequency of contact	One-to-one contact, increased access to student on a shift-by-shift basis.	Defined in terms of relationship but commonly 1 hour per fortnight or as dictated by need between clinical supervisor and supervisee.	Defined by the mentor and mentee, often in response to professional development needs.
Aims of relationship	To ensure smooth transition from student to competent practitioner.	Increase therapeutic skills. Provide support for clinicians in their professional life.	To guide the mentee through career development over a period of time. Developing leadership qualities. Transition of values and beliefs.
Primary focus of relationship	Role modelling, professional socialisation, orientation, educational and supportive. Student assessment.	Multiple, includes organisational, professional and personal objectives.	Career progression, professional development, more closely aligned with clinical supervision, although not formalised.
Facilitator	In-house nurse, clinically active in workplace. Familiar with clinical setting.	Experienced, trained clinician often from within supervisee's agency. Can be independent, external supervisor of a number of disciplines.	Usually from within supervisee's agency. However, may be located in different agency as relationship progresses over years.
Potential benefits	Learning is 'real' and has increased meaning. One-to-one relationship. Develops clinical skills and application of theory to practice. Benefits for preceptors, agency. Promotion of profession recruitment and retention.	Learn, improve and refine clinical skills. Enhance reflective practice. Identify issues related to transference and counter-transference.	Long-term 'wise counsellor' role. Able to follow mentee's career development over longer period regardless of where mentor is located.
Limitations	Workloads can interfere with learning. Mismatched relationship. Evaluation in isolation, inadequate preceptor preparation. Preceptor burnout.	Availability of appropriately prepared clinical supervisors. Cost can be prohibitive.	Lacks formalised, clear structure. Issues/focus may be driven more by experience of mentor to the detriment of mentee's independence.

Adapted from Charleston *et al.* (2002).

development, support, growth and learning, as well as of personal support.

Common concepts of clinical supervision include:

- Clinical supervision is a supportive space for professional reflection which promotes growth, development and learning.
- The relationship between the supervisor and the supervisee is paramount and at all times will affect the outcome of clinical supervision.
- Clinical supervision needs to be voluntary and all parties involved in supervision need to be committed, open and honest.

Reflective exercise

- Brainstorm some of the words that describe clinical supervision.
- From these words begin forming a definition of clinical supervision.
- Consider the key stakeholders in your organisation. Would the definition you have developed be an acceptable definition of clinical supervision from their perspective?

You might want to conduct this exercise with some of the key stakeholders in your organisation – together you may find a definition that aptly describes clinical supervision from multiple perspectives, and possibly reach a compromise that is acceptable to all.

Table 1.3 Clinical supervision – comparisons with other forums.

Forums	Similarities	Differences
Handover		
Case reviews or clinical case conferences		
Supervision of new graduate nurses		
Education sessions/programs		
Peer support		
Critical incident debriefing		
Employee assistance/support programs		
Mediation		

Table 1.4 Comparison of other forums/professional relationships in your organisation with clinical supervision.

Forums	Similarities	Differences

Table 1.5   Clinical supervision – comparisons with other forums (suggestions).

Forums	Similarities	Differences
Handover	The clinical handover is focused on the patient and clinical/work-related issues, handovers are intended to be non-judgemental, objective and supportive. Handovers, like clinical supervision, present a way to convey information from one nurse to another about a particular patient or clinical scenario.	Unlike clinical supervision, handovers are extremely time limited, there is often considerable pressure for handover to be brief, only highlighting the most pertinent clinical information. The main focus of the handover is objective information sharing, rather than exploring the subjective and the relationship through offering or allowing time to reflect on the patient's clinical care or the nurses' clinical decision making. The primary focus is on the patient not the clinician or the clinician–patient interaction.
Case reviews or clinical case conferences	The focus in clinical reviews and case conferences is the clinical work and like clinical supervision there is often time allowed for guided reflection on the clinical work and time allowed to explore clinical issues in much more detail than that of a clinical handover.	In a case conference the focus is on clients and their treatment, not on the clinician and the clinician–patient relationship. There are usually multiple clinicians in attendance and involved at a clinical review/case conference and often there are time pressures with a number of patients needing to be reviewed in one meeting.
Supervision of new graduate nurses	Similar to clinical supervision the graduate year supervision provided by nurses is supportive, educational and focused on assisting a nurse to develop specific clinical/ therapeutic skills.	The supervision offered in graduate year is time limited, usually only for the duration of the graduate year. The supervision is often compulsory and many supervisees do not have capacity to choose the supervisor. The main goal is to assist the graduate during his or her first year of practice and may include an assessment component.
Education sessions/programs	Education sessions and programs are supportive, educational and focused on assisting the nurse to develop specific clinical/therapeutic skills.	Unlike clinical supervision the focus in educational issues is on specific topics (as chosen by the educator or the organisation). These sessions are time limited and designed to meet the needs of many and not the individual.

Continued

Table 1.5 *Continued*

Forums	Similarities	Differences
Peer support	Peer support programs are usually voluntary and self-initiated. They are supportive, educational and focused on assisting peers to develop specific clinical/therapeutic skills.	Peer support is often an informal process, whereas clinical supervision is formal. Peer support is focused on bringing together peers who work in close proximity, usually the same team. Unlike clinical supervision there is not a designated leader or clinical supervisor – the peers provide each other with mutual support, or leadership can be rotated within the group.
Critical incident debriefing	Critical incident debriefing, like clinical supervision, can be offered individually or to a group. The focus is on providing a supportive, non-judgemental forum for the nurses to explore a particular clinical event/situation. There is no assessment involved.	The focus of critical incident debriefing is purely on supporting staff through the trauma of a specific event. It is short term and there is little or no choice of the facilitator.
Employee assistance/support programs	Many employees offer variations of employee assistance programs. Generally these programs are established to provide support for staff on work issues. It is a confidential process that is offered by the employer during work time.	Most employee assistance programs are short term and funded by the employer. They can be accessed anonymously and personal as well as professional/work issues can be discussed.
Mediation	Mediation, like supervision, should be offered by an experienced and well-trained clinician. The focus is on supporting staff during a particular clinical or work-related event. The process is non-judgemental and often confidential. Generally, it is intended to be a voluntary process.	Mediation involves working with two or more people on a specific event or incident. There is often no choice about who conducts the mediation session and sometimes participants may not feel they have a choice about being involved.

Again the 1990s in the UK and Europe provide us with most of the commonly accepted and utilised definitions of clinical supervision, for example:

> *Clinical supervision can be defined as didactic and supported method for reflection, which has the potential to encourage and enhance nurses' professional development and personal growth.* (Severinsson, 1999: 23)

The UK Central Council for Nursing, Midwifery and Health Visiting defined clinical supervision as:

> *A formal process of professional support and learning which enables individual practitioners to develop knowledge and competence, assume responsibility for their own practice and enhance consumer protection and safety of care in complex clinical situations. It is central to the process of learning and to the scope of the expansion of practice and should be seen as a means of encouraging self-assessment and analytical and reflective skills.* (UK Central Council for Nursing, Midwifery and Health Visiting, 1995: 3)

For the purposes of this book the following definition of clinical supervision by Hancox & Lynch (2002: 6) will be used:

> *Clinical supervision is a formal process of consultation between two or more professionals. The focus is to provide support for the supervisee(s) in order to promote self awareness, professional development and growth within the context of their professional environment.*

Along with the generally accepted components of a definition it is important to highlight the formal nature of the relationship and acknowledge both individual and group clinical supervision rather than limiting a definition to one or the other.

Benefits of clinical supervision

The stressful working conditions nurses frequently face have been emphasised as a major factor contributing to nurses leaving the profession. Most recently this has been highlighted in National Review of Nursing Education (Commonwealth of Australia, 2002) and the Senate Inquiry into Nursing (Senate Select Committee on Mental Health, 2006), both undertaken on behalf of the Commonwealth of Australia. Surprisingly, however, these reports did not consider clinical supervision as a potential strategy for minimising stress in the workplace.

However, the Nurse Recruitment and Retention Committee in Victoria (Department of Human Services, Victoria, 2001) stated that as a high priority:

> . . . *clinical supervision for registered nurses be introduced into the public health system as a strategy for retaining experienced, qualified nurses in clinical settings and that each nurse, regardless of full-time or part-time status, will receive two hours per month of clinical supervision time.*

Clinical supervision in Australia

Clinical supervision in the mental health field is not a new concept. Disciplines such as psychology and social work have a strong tradition with this initiative. For example, clinical supervision is a mandatory requirement for registration as a psychologist. By working alongside these other health professionals, many mental health nurses have seen the advantages of, and have sought, clinical supervision. However, this tended to occur on an ad hoc and individual basis, rather than as part of a broader professional or organisational culture.

More recently, other specialties of nursing and midwifery are acknowledging the benefits of clinical supervision for their practice and ultimately for improving the quality of patient care. However, the development of clinical supervision in Australia could be best described as patchy. While no doubt there is important work being undertaken, this appears to be inconsistent and isolated. In conducting the background research for this book, contact was made with the all of the known national nursing organisations in Australia. Those who responded to the request for information indicated that they had no policies or position statements in relation to clinical supervision for nurses. The fact that this term is not well understood became obvious as part of this process. The responses from many of the organisations clearly identified confusion with supervised practice for nurses returning to the nursing workforce after a lengthy period of absence, or the supervision of students or new graduates.

At the government level specific policies have been developed in Victoria and Western Australia. The Department of Human Services, Victoria (2006) released a brief document which despite being titled as guidelines could be more appropriately described as a philosophical overview supporting the benefits of clinical supervision for nurses. Rather than providing guidance, the document delegated the responsibility for selecting and developing models of clinical supervision to individual mental health services (this document is discussed in further detail in Chapter 3).

The Victorian Government provided some leadership in clinical supervision following the Enterprise Bargaining Agreement of August

2000. The Department of Human Services, Mental Health Branch announced the injection of considerable funds to support mental health nursing within the state. The introduction of clinical supervision into all mental health services was identified as an important strategy in both encouraging professional development and providing much needed support for nursing. While there is significant anecdotal evidence to suggest that clinical supervision is now better understood and more available as a result of this initiative, the absence of formalised guidelines and systematic evaluation makes it difficult to estimate how successful the implementation of clinical supervision has been.

A considerably more comprehensive framework was produced by the Department of Health, Western Australia (2005). This document defines and presents an overview of the value of clinical supervision, delineates the roles of supervisor and supervisee, suggests some preferred models of supervision and describes how the supervisory relationship should be initiated and developed. Ethical issues and procedural matters (such as how to deal with conflict should it emerge) are addressed. Examples of supervision agreements, schedules and record notes are included. However, it does not address the broader issue of how clinical supervision can be implemented.

The activity around clinical supervision in the mental health area has also occurred within other states and territories of Australia, although these efforts appear to reflect clinical and academic leadership rather than government direction. Again, this indicates the absence of systematic evaluation and a clear structure to enable the experiences of others to be shared and learned from.

Communications with nurses with direct involvement (either past or current) with the implementation of clinical supervision for nurses suggest the process has not been carefully considered, planned and/or evaluated. In some cases significant amounts of money have been invested in the education and training of clinical supervisors and supervisees. While positive outcomes have been observed at the anecdotal level, sustainability has been an issue, and many initiatives have not continued beyond the early implementation stages.

Recognition of the importance of clinical supervision is not reflected in the Australian nursing literature. An article published in 2006 (White & Roche, 2006: 217) notes that the use of clinical supervision in Australia remains underdeveloped. This research, undertaken in New South Wales with a sample of 601 nurses across 17 mental health services, confirmed this view by finding that more than two-thirds of the sample were not currently receiving clinical supervision and concluded that mental health nursing '. . . has yet to engage clinical supervision in a systematically coherent manner.'

Before clinical supervision can be implemented on a wide scale, its meaning must become more clearly understood and its potential value appreciated. A primary aim of this book is to provide a systematic overview of clinical supervision ranging from a clear understanding of what clinical supervision is, through implementation, the relevant legal and ethical issues, and ultimately to a detailed exploration of the supervisory relationship and processes. It is a book written by Australian nurses with clinical and academic interest and expertise in the area, for Australian nurses, whom we hope will find this work useful in their quest to understand and implement clinical supervision in a wide range of clinical areas, with a systematic and sustainable approach.

The contents in detail

Chapter 2: Practice development in nursing

As a practice-based profession, the articulation, development and improvement of practice must remain at the forefront. This chapter presents an important theoretical underpinning of this book. The importance of practice development and the significant inter-relationship we recognise between practice development and clinical supervision are presented. More specifically this chapter will:

* define practice development
* consider the importance of practice development for nursing
* articulate the contribution of clinical supervision to practice development.

Chapter 3: Implementing clinical supervision

The implementation of clinical supervision cannot occur in a vacuum. Every health care service has its own unique culture that comprises specific characteristics that will either support or resist the introduction of clinical supervision. A systematic and rigorous approach is therefore required in order that clinical supervision becomes a reality. More specifically this chapter:

* introduces the importance of a structured implementation strategy
* explores the importance of organisational culture to the implementation of clinical supervision
* provides an overview of the implementation of clinical supervision within one health service
* presents a research-based model designed to guide the implementation process
* explores role definition and meaning, the impact of role and the link to culture within organisations.

Chapter 4: Approaches to clinical supervision

When it comes to clinical supervision it is not a case of 'one-size fits all'. The aim of this chapter is to provide a brief overview of different approaches to the provision of supervision. More specifically this chapter:

- distinguishes between individual and group clinical supervision
- considers the implications for the use of individual vs group clinical supervision
- considers the advantages and disadvantages of external and internal clinical supervision
- discusses the relative advantages and disadvantages of multidisciplinary vs discipline-specific clinical supervision.

Chapter 5: Models for clinical supervision

As a formal process, clinical supervision requires a structured interaction between two (or more) individuals that is directed towards the achievement of specific outcomes. Models have been developed specifically for clinical supervision; however, some supervisors prefer to adapt other therapeutic or nursing models for use in this environment. The aim of this chapter is to:

- illustrate the importance of models for clinical supervision
- provide an overview of models commonly used in clinical supervision.

It is not possible to cover all possible models in this chapter but a brief introduction to the following models is provided:

- psychoanalytic
- systems psychodynamics
- reflective practice
- Kadushin
- Proctor
- Peplau
- solution focused.

Chapter 6: Legal and ethical issues in clinical supervision

Nursing is an intensely personal profession. Nurses engage with patients at an extremely vulnerable time in their lives. Many ethical issues and dilemmas arise in this context and, like other professionals, nurses are required to practice within a legal and ethical framework. Clinical supervision is similarly personal and encompasses a range of ethical issues. There is, however, no specific legislation that pertains to clinical supervision. However, broader legal principles are relevant to this practice. The aim of this chapter is to:

- provide a brief overview of the Australian legal system
- discuss the legal implications for clinical supervision, duty of care, negligence and vicarious liability
- consider the implications of dual relationships within clinical supervision
- discuss the importance of confidentiality
- consider ethical issues and ethical dilemmas
- consider the issue of mandatory vs voluntary participation in clinical supervision.

Chapter 7: Enhancing the supervisory relationship: the roles of the supervisor and supervisee

The aim of this chapter is to explore the roles of clinical supervisor and supervisee and consider the factors that must be achieved in order to strengthen these roles and therefore enhance the supervisory relationship. More specifically the contents of this chapter include:

- the necessary skills and knowledge to provide supervision
- what the supervisor needs to know about the supervisee
- the importance of education and training
- supervisor burnout, what it is and how to avoid it
- establishing boundaries for safe practice
- the importance of self-awareness and reflection
- choosing the right supervisor for you
- what the supervisee needs to know about the supervisor
- making the most of clinical supervision
- education and training for supervisees
- dealing with problems in the supervisory relationship.

Chapter 8: Clinical supervision in action

Clinical supervision is about much more than a couple of people in a room chatting. It is an important relationship that must be taken seriously if it is to fulfil its promise. The aim of this chapter is to provide guidance in preparing for the establishment of a supervisory relationship, including:

- the Hancox/Lynch model of clinical supervision
- the development of clinical supervision agreements
- how to conduct the first session
- conducting subsequent clinical supervision sessions.

Chapter 9: Evaluating clinical supervision

The key to the sustainability of clinical supervision lies in the ability to produce evidence to show that it makes a difference. That evidence will only come through systematic evaluation. The aim of this chapter is to discuss:

- the importance of evaluation
- what evaluation is and how it differs from research
- different types of evaluation
- what should be evaluated
- an overview of methodologies for evaluation
- approaches to measuring impact, including financial, job satisfaction and consumer outcomes
- recommendations for future research.

Conclusion

In this chapter the reader has been introduced to the concept of clinical supervision. It is hoped that this has dispelled some of the common misconceptions and provided clarity by distinguishing clinical supervision from other supervisory and therapeutic relationships. The importance of clinical supervision for nurses and for nursing has been described. Finally, an overview of the structure and contents of this book has been provided.

References

Charleston, R., Hancox, K. & Lynch, L. (2002) *Preceptorship in Psychiatric Nursing, Course Materials*. Melbourne: Centre for Psychiatric Nursing Research and Practice.

Commonwealth of Australia (2002) *National Review of Nursing Education 2002: Our Duty of Care*. Canberra: Department of Education Science and Training.

Consedine, M. (1994) *Taking the next step: The selection, development and training of nurses to provide supervision for role development in mental health nursing. Proceedings of the 20th Annual Convention of the Australian and New Zealand College of Mental Health Nurses*. Brisbane: Australian and New Zealand College of Mental Health Nurses, pp 504–515.

Department of Health, Western Australia (2005) *Clinical Supervision: A Framework for WA Mental Health Services and Clinicians*. Perth: Department of Health.

Department of Human Services, Victoria (2001) *Nurse Recruitment and Retention Committee – Final Report, May 2001*. Melbourne: Department of Human Services.

Department of Human Services, Victoria (2006) *Guidelines for Clinical Supervision*. Victoria: Department of Human Services. Retrieved from www.dhs.vic.gov.au/mentalhealth, February 2007.

Hancox, K. & Lynch, L. (2002) *Clinical Supervision for Health Care Professionals. Course Guide*. Carlton, Victoria: University of Melbourne and the Centre for Psychiatric Nursing Research and Practice.

Mackereth, P. (1996) Clinical supervision for potent practice. *Complementary Therapies in Nursing & Midwifery*, 3, 38–41.

Moores, Y. (1994) Chief Nursing Officer (CNO) Professional Letter (94:5) Clinical Supervision. London: Department of Health.

Senate Select Committee on Mental Health (2006) *A National Approach to Mental Health – From Crisis to Community*. Canberra: Commonwealth of Australia.

Severinsson, E. (1999) Ethics in clinical supervision – an introduction to the theory and practice of different supervision models. *Collegian*, 6, 23–28.

Simms, J. (1993) Supervision. In: Wright, H. & Giddley, M. (eds). *Mental Health Nursing*. London: Chapman & Hall.

UK Central Council for Nursing, Midwifery and Health Visiting (1995) *Position Statement on Clinical Supervision for Nursing and Health Visiting*. Annex 1 to registrar's letter 4/1995. London: NMC, pp 1–5.

White, E. & Roche, M. (2006) A selective review of mental health nursing in New South Wales, Australia, in relation to clinical supervision. *International Journal of Mental Health Nursing*, 15, 209–219.

Yegdich, T. (1999) Clinical supervision and managerial supervision: some historical and conceptual considerations. *Journal of Advanced Nursing*, 30(5), 1195–1204.

Practice development in nursing

Introduction

From the definitions explored in Chapter 1, it is very clear that the aim, intent and purpose of clinical supervision are to bring about an increased understanding and the ongoing development of nursing practice. The link between clinical supervision and practice development is therefore obvious. Given that one aim of this book is to provide a framework to assist with the introduction, implementation and 'doing' of clinical supervision within a safe and supportive environment, a discussion of practice development is essential.

The specific aims of this chapter are to:

- define practice development
- consider the importance of practice development for nursing
- articulate the contribution of clinical supervision to practice development.

This chapter is intended as background for clinical supervision. It is not a guide to introduce practice development, but rather seeks to explore the important inter-relationship between practice development and clinical supervision.

Stacey's story

I always wanted to be a nurse. As a child I spent several months in and out of hospital following a serious car accident and I learned how important nurses are. They were like my parents, teachers and friends all rolled into one. Thinking about how much they meant to me, I wanted to make this kind of difference to other people.

Continued

I graduated 10 years ago and have been working in a large metropolitan hospital; I have worked in a number of medical and surgical units. Once I registered as a nurse I came to respect the nurses who had cared for me even more because I understood some of the difficulties of the job I had not seen from the other side. Busy workloads, staff shortages, piles of paper work, doing more with less, and dealing with the competing demands of patient care and hospital bureaucracy at times have made my job feel impossible. I am sure it was the same for the nurses who looked after me, but they never seemed to show it.

I still love nursing but I am constantly faced with the challenges and shortcomings of nursing as a profession and of me as a nurse. From the time I start my shift I barely have time to think beyond responding to the needs and demands of the patients I am caring for. Even then I often feel I am not doing my job properly. I often go home knowing I could have done more, thinking about Mr Jones and his family, very anxious about his major cardiac surgery and how I had to cut short the time I spent talking to them because Mrs Davis had returned from surgery and Miss Hanson was vomiting profusely.

At times I think there must be a better way to do things, where patient care and nurse satisfaction are both improved, where patient care really is more important than completing paper work, where nurses have the time to read up on the latest developments in their areas of expertise, where professional development opportunities are available and prioritised. The frustrations I and many of my colleagues experience are frequently blamed on funding and staffing. No doubt that is true but I still sometimes wonder if we use those things as an excuse for feeling powerless, that we should learn to live with our frustrations and make the best of our situations rather than trying to change things. Not that we should not strive for improved resources and staffing but that we should not let these external factors be the prime drivers of our professional practice.

I have raised my concerns in staff meetings. I do not think these views are welcomed by the nurse unit manager, perhaps he sees what I am saying as a criticism of his skills and abilities of a manager. It is not meant to be. Looking at a different way of doing things cannot be the responsibility of one person alone, it should be a team activity. Some of my colleagues have told me privately that they agree with me. Others say that there is not enough time in the day to do what we are already required to do, let alone do any more. I also know of many nurses who have left nursing, and many others who are considering doing the same, because they feel their job is more about putting out spot fires than making a real difference to people's lives.

I think it is a shame that we consider effective, person-centred nursing care as an extra burden in a busy job. I still think that somehow as a team we could find a way to do stop, look, think and to do things better, but I just don't know where to start.

Nursing and practice development

Stacey's story is 'kind of' fictitious. We say 'kind of' because as nurses ourselves we can relate to Stacey through our individual experiences and those of the many nurses we have worked with as clinicians, managers, educators and academics, in a broad range of specialty areas ranging from general medical–surgical, palliative care, midwifery, rehabilitation and mental health, across the life span from birth to death and across a broad range of geographical settings.

I am sure you, the reader, can relate to Stacey's story and the difficulties she experienced in meeting the demands that appeared to come from all angles, and often seemed to distract her from the very thing that attracted her to nursing in the first place: the ability to make a difference in the lives of people as they recover from illness or injury.

Stacey's story has been included in this chapter because we believe she is alluding to the need for the unit where she works to adopt practice development principles in order to work towards a more responsive, patient-oriented culture, and create an environment that also provides a greater sense of achievement and job satisfaction for nurses, rather than becoming quietly accepting and despondent about the way things are.

Clinical supervision could be an important resource in assisting Stacey to achieve her goals. For example, group supervision could provide an opportunity for Stacey and her colleagues to discuss and reflect on their work environment, and together they may be able to find ways to do things differently. They may arrive at some strategies to change their practice and as a group can provide much needed support to raise their ideas with their manager.

More specifically, Stacey noticed that the way patient care was allocated seemed to make it more difficult to spend time with her patients. There did not seem to be much continuity with patients, and nurses seemed to be allocated different patients on just about every shift. This meant that more time was spent becoming familiar with the patients, their needs and their circumstances. Stacey's colleagues agreed that it would save time if they aimed to work with the same patients where possible.

Group clinical supervision could provide an important venue for Stacey and her colleagues to find a way to suggest a new approach to the unit manager without him feeling attacked or that his authority was being questioned. As individuals, Stacey and the other nurses may feel powerless and reluctant to approach their manager, whereas collectively they can find mutual support and develop strategies to introduce the subject in a way that is more likely to be heard.

What is practice development?

There is considerable divergence in the literature regarding what practice development is, and therefore how it should be defined. A broadly accepted definition is presented by Garbett & McCormack (2002: 88):

> . . . *a continuous process of improvement towards increased effectiveness in patient centred care. This is brought about by helping healthcare teams to develop their knowledge and skills and to transform the culture and context of care. It is enabled and supported by facilitators committed to a systematic, rigorous continuous process of emancipatory change that reflects the perspectives of service users.*

While it is not the focus of this chapter to debate the various definitions provided, it is important to emphasise some aspects of the Garbett and McCormack definition, particularly that clinical supervision:

- is a continuous process
- is a transformative process
- requires facilitation
- involves the perspectives of service users.

The meaning and importance of these factors will now be considered.

Continuous

We are all aware of the dynamic nature of health care delivery. Factors such as advances in technology and medical science, and social, political and economic forces continually challenge nurses and other health professionals to strive towards improvement of health care within a financially constrained environment. Practice development does not therefore represent a problem that can be solved and completed. Practice change is inevitable, and a practice development approach ensures that change is not haphazard or reactionary but rather an ongoing process.

Transformative

The changing of practice within health care is often aimed at specific tasks. For example, a health service may identify that admission procedures are lengthy and result in considerable delay in transferring patients to the appropriate ward or unit. Emergency departments are frequently overcrowded and patients and their families are distressed by patients having to remain on trolleys in a congested and chaotic environment for longer than they need to.

The task or project approach to overcoming this problem would involve focusing on the specifics. For example, the current admission procedures would be examined in detail. By mapping the patient journey through admission and exploring each specific part of the journey, one can begin to form a view of what admission practices assist and which practices impede patient admissions. Then alternatives would be sought either from existing practices from other institutions or through developing and trialling an alternative model. The problem may be resolved in the short term, but longer-term change is unlikely unless a thorough exploration and understanding of the culture and context of the organisation is grasped, so people come to appreciate what contributed to the original problem.

Facilitated change

Effective and sustainable practice development will not happen of its own accord, and although commitment and desire are important ingredients to effect change and development, on their own they are insufficient. Changing and improving practice must be facilitated. It must be coordinated, driven and maintained. The practice development facilitator therefore represents a crucial role that must be considered and nurtured if the process is to be successful.

Despite acknowledging the importance of facilitation, little attention has been paid to the facilitation role in the literature (McCormack *et al.*, 2004). However, the themes identified from the literature and from interviews with persons occupying a facilitation role (McCormack & Garbett, 2002; Rycroft-Malone, 2004) suggest that the facilitator or practice development nurse, however named, must possess a range of skills and attributes that will enhance the role of encouraging organisational change from both top–down and bottom–up perspectives.

The concept of facilitation is a pivotal part of this definition in demonstrating the close relationship between clinical supervision and practice development and will therefore be considered in greater detail in a later section of this chapter.

Involving service users

The right and opportunity for the users or consumers of services to become actively involved in the planning, delivery and evaluation of health care services is increasingly becoming an expectation of contemporary health care. In Australia this expectation is now enshrined in policy in the mental health field (Commonwealth of Australia, 1997, 1998, 2003), but has not received this level of acknowledgement within the general health care system.

Although consumer participation is a part of mental health policy, there is evidence to suggest a lack of translation into practice (Lammers & Happell, 2004; Goodwin & Happell, 2006). Consumer participation is frequently described as tokenistic, with limited evidence to support its effective and widespread incorporation into service structures.

The Garbett and McCormack (2002) definition clearly indicates that practice development should be oriented towards patient-centred care and that it should reflect the perspectives of service users.

If the facilitation role receives little attention in the literature, user involvement receives even less. The edited book by McCormack *et al.* (2004), considered by many as the 'bible' of practice development, devotes a significant proportion of a chapter to facilitation but only short snippets address consumer involvement. Given that the improvement of patient care is at the centre of practice development, this represents a significant and regrettable omission.

If the aim of practice development is to improve health care outcomes for those who use services, then it is imperative that patients are included at all stages of the process.

Evidence-based practice

Much of what we take for granted in nursing practice tends to rely more on routine and ritual than on the findings of systematic research (Hutchinson & Johnston, 2006). It is fair to say that nurses have an ambivalent relationship with research. On the one hand they acknowledge its value and importance, while on the other hand they question its accessibility and relevance for contemporary health care practice.

More specifically, some major barriers to evidence-based practice have been identified:

- Nurses do not know about it. Access to resources such as the internet or the appropriate journals where the relevant research can be located can be problematic.
- Nurses do not know how to do it. Nurses often feel they lack the necessary expertise required to both find the literature through systematic searching and appraise the scientific merit and relevance of available research literature.
- Nurses do not have time for it. The high workloads and acuity levels within current clinical practice mean that nurses often do not have the time to access, appraise and implement relevant research findings.
- Nurses do not have adequate access to computers or quiet space for reading and reflection.

Evidence-based practice is not primarily about becoming a researcher, but rather about becoming a consumer of research, using the research that has already been conducted to find new and different ways of doing things (or provide justification for the existing ones) that have been demonstrated to have successful outcomes, rather than doing the same things 'because it has always been done this way' or 'it feels good this way'. Evidence-based practice challenges the age-old saying, 'If it ain't broke why fix it?' by suggesting that merely seeming to be effective is not a good enough reason to maintain a particular practice when there may be an approach that has been proven to be more successful.

Evidence-based practice relies on a hierarchy of evidence where the randomised-controlled trial is considered to represent the best available evidence and expert opinion, and, while it is still regarded as evidence, qualitative research is considered to be the least rigorous and convincing evidence. Understandably, clinicians frequently criticise evidence-based practice for not placing higher value on the knowledge and skills that are derived from practice.

In considering the nature and potential value of evidence-based practice, the parallels with practice development are clearly apparent. Both encourage self-reflection and enquiry in order to develop and improve nursing practice for the benefit of the recipients of our services. In order to be successful, both require a significant culture change where nurses are prepared to look beyond the way things have always been done, indeed to question and challenge existing practices, in order to find better ways to practice.

Given the identified barriers, in order for evidence-based practice to become part of nursing teams or units, support and leadership are required. Not only the expertise, but also the dedicated time to access and appraise literature is necessary. Rycroft-Malone (2004) described the need for a facilitator who is sufficiently skilled and knowledgeable to assist nurses 'to make sense of the evidence' (p. 135):

> . . . *facilitation refers to a process of enabling individuals and groups to understand the processes they have to go through to change aspects of their behaviour or attitudes to themselves, their work or other individuals.*
> (Rycroft-Malone, 2004: 136)

Once a team has made sense of the evidence and appreciates its relevance to the practice setting, the role of the facilitator is to guide the implementation process. It is one thing to recognise the need for change, but the process of making it happen can be particularly challenging. This may require the alteration of age-old practices, and mean significant changes to nurses' roles. Without skilled facilitation, the temptation to slip back into the way things have always been may be difficult to resist.

The importance of practice development

As a practice-based profession, nursing has a commitment to the articulation, development and improvement of clinical practice in order to ensure that the highest standard of care and treatment is provided for the patients of health services.

Historically, there was a tendency to view nursing knowledge as that gained from books or in the classroom, as distinct from nursing experience, which was that gained through exposure to the practice setting. One author clearly remembers that during the lead-up to her state final examinations, she was told (by more than one nurse educator): 'You now know more than you will ever know'. This statement sent chills through the spines of anxious nursing students who considered the idea of becoming a 'sister' with fear and trepidation because they felt they knew very little and were apprehensive about the expectations that would soon be upon them. The students distinguished between the knowledge they needed to pass the examinations and the knowledge they needed to practice effectively as registered nurses.

Apart from scaring nursing students at a stressful period in their careers, the statement, if taken literally, pays little respect to the knowledge and skills that are derived from and embedded in nursing practice. Knowledge is seen to be theoretical knowledge and final year students know most because they have learned it recently and have crammed their brains full of all this knowledge in case it is needed in the exam.

More recently, the appreciation of what is learned and developed in the clinical setting has increasingly come to be regarded not just as experience but as knowledge in its own right. The relationship between practice and theory should therefore not be seen as one way, with theory dictating or determining practice. Rather, the relationship should be seen as dynamic and continually changing, with theory being influenced by practice as much as it influences it. Practice therefore should both contribute to and be influenced by theoretical knowledge.

The recent popularity of practice development reflects broader influences over contemporary health care, including:

- accountability
- person-centred care.

Accountability

Economic constraints continually place pressure on health services and health professionals to demonstrate how they contribute to effective health care outcomes in a cost-effective manner. A systematic approach to practice development potentially provides a framework for articulating the relationship between specific practices and health or service outcomes.

As the cost of nursing services increases and ongoing problems with recruitment and retention are evident, nursing is likely to be called to account for the value and importance of the contribution it makes to health care. The resulting arguments need to be about more than the tasks associated with nursing work. Considerable support is already evident for the so-called generic or third-level personnel to take on the less technical aspects of patient care traditionally considered important functions of nursing, such as meeting hygiene needs. Practice development must become an important strategy if nursing is to continue to be recognised as a profession that positively influences health care well beyond its component parts or tasks.

Person-centred care

Many health professionals find the suggestion that services need to become person centred a curious concept. After all, is not the primary purpose of health care services to provide care and treatment for those experiencing health care problems? Providing care and treatment is of course an important consideration, but we can all appreciate the many bureaucratic processes inherent within the modern health care system that at times mean that policies and procedures dictate the approach to the care provided rather than the specific needs of individual service users. While policies and procedures are developed to enhance quality or ensure safety, for example, there are times when the processes appear to become ends in themselves rather than the means to promote the ultimate end of patient-centred care.

Reflective exercise

Consider the organisation/unit/team you work within and reflect on:

- the amount of time spent completing tasks that do not involve direct interaction with patients
- the extent to which nursing practice follows a specific routine
- the extent to which these routines can be justified in the best interests of service users rather than to promote the smooth functioning of the unit for the benefit of staff
- the frequency of being unable to attend to specific legitimate needs of service users because of priority needing to be given to organisational imperatives
- the extent to which the health outcomes you identify as desirable reflect your views of what is in the best interest of the patients rather than the patients' view of what is in their best interests.

As a result of these reflections we are confident you will agree that at times the processes, policies and procedures designed to enhance service delivery can distract attention from meeting the needs of individuals to meeting the requirements of the broader system. While we are not suggesting for a moment that policies and procedures are not an essential part of health care delivery, we would suggest that some bureaucratic processes can seem unduly cumbersome and therefore divert attention from patient care. Patient-centred care, we would argue, is not an automatic feature of contemporary health care services but rather one which requires a concentrated and concerted approach. Practice development presents a model that enhances that approach.

The development of patient-centred care requires a commitment to encouraging and facilitating the active involvement of service users in health care delivery both on an individual and on a systemic basis. On an individual basis this requires a practice environment that moves away from routines and bureaucratic processes to create an environment where patient needs are the primary focus. Patients or consumers (as they are more commonly known in the mental health field) are encouraged to move beyond the passive role, which defers to the expertise and judgement of health professionals, and become actively involved.

The importance of practice development in this approach may be more complex than it first appears. Encouraging active participation in individual care requires a lot more than just words describing a new idea. Traditionally, health service delivery has relied quite heavily on routines. One author recalls that as a student nurse admitting patients to a medical ward she would ask new patients whether they preferred a shower or a bath and the time of day they preferred to attend to their hygiene. Unfortunately, it was nothing more than a paper exercise; no matter how they answered the question all patients were showered as early as possible in the morning to ensure the showers were completed by 10.00 am. Facilitating consumer participation involves much more than just asking questions; it means actively responding to patients as representing the centre of treatment.

Practice development and professional development

Despite the inter-relationship between the two, practice development and professional development are separate concepts and need to be distinguished in order that a clear understanding of practice development is achieved. Professional development pertains to individual nurses, and the process for attaining the knowledge and skills they require to practice effectively. It generally constitutes one of three main activities:

(1) self-directed learning through reading journals and other scholarly publications
(2) attending short courses or conferences
(3) formal postgraduate studies.

Practice development, on the other hand, describes the process where the outcomes gained through professional development are translated into actual practice and result in improved health outcomes for service users.

Example

Family-sensitive practice

Professional development: Jenny, a registered nurse from a paediatric unit, undertakes a training course on family-sensitive practice. She gains considerable knowledge and skill about meeting the needs of families of hospitalised children and how to facilitate their active involvement in the care and treatment of their loved one. This new knowledge is likely to positively influence Jenny's nursing practice in relation to families, but the impact on the unit as a whole will generally be minimal without a broader practice development framework.

Practice development: On completing the family-sensitive practice course, Jenny consults with Vanessa, the practice development nurse on her unit. Jenny's initial professional development experience evolves into practice development through the following process:

- Jenny and Vanessa discuss the importance of introducing a more family-sensitive approach to the way the unit operates.
- Initially Vanessa and Jenny work together, with the support and approval of the unit manager, to access literature and identify other paediatric units that have adopted this framework. Evidence-based practice is an important part of this process. A review of the literature on family-sensitive practice is crucial as a starting point. The literature must then be appraised and considered according to both the quality of the research and its relevance to the particular paediatric unit.
- After analysing and synthesising the information they have collected, Jenny and Vanessa present an overview of family-sensitive practice to the broader team. This involves a critical appraisal of the best available evidence.
- The process of introducing family-sensitive practice begins as a team process using an action-oriented and reflective process. As the practice development nurse, Vanessa observes and notes the responses of nurses to the idea of developing their practice in this new direction. She identifies those who are likely to champion the cause or at least actively support the initiative. She identifies those who appear to be resistant to, or are struggling with, the idea and offers her support and expertise accordingly.
- Vanessa identifies the educational and professional development needs of the unit staff. For example, would other nurses benefit from attending the course Jenny completed? Should all staff attend? Is sufficient funding available to support this level of attendance? If not, what decision-making process will determine which nurses are selected to attend? What are the nurses' needs in relation to evidence-based practice? Do they need to learn how to locate, retrieve and appraise research evidence? Although Vanessa may play the leading role, it is important that these skills are also developed amongst members of the team.

Continued

- Although the implementation of a family-sensitive approach as a practice development initiative is a team responsibility, Vanessa has an important role in providing support and encouragement, in keeping the team on track and in seeking the resources required.
- Vanessa holds regular meetings with the team to consider progress, barriers and other issues that might affect the advancement of the initiative. She considers the most appropriate approaches to evaluating the initiative. The regular meetings held with the team form part of the evaluation process as their feedback is integrated and the project grows and develops. Patient feedback is sought either via invitation to small focus groups or through the feedback forms completed on discharge. Where successful outcomes are demonstrated, the practice is more likely to be accepted by the team itself and by the health care administration. This is essential if the ongoing commitment to provide resources is to be secured.

Professional development: Other nurses with a recognised key role in the implementation of family-sensitive practice undertake the course originally completed by Jenny. Jenny and Vanessa facilitate a professional development session for staff on what has been learned to date.

Practice development: Vanessa organises regular meetings of the nurses who have completed the family-sensitive course. In these meetings they:

- identify practices and aspects of the ward culture that may not operate in the best interests of families
- consider the strategies necessary to ensure these practices become more family sensitive
- plan the interventions that will be necessary to implement the identified strategies
- anticipate potential barriers (e.g. staff resistance, hospital policies and funding) that might impede the implementation process and consider the resources required to overcome these barriers
- constantly evaluate and reassess the progress of the initiatives and what further work needs to be done to reach the goal
- develop strategies to ensure family-sensitive practices are embedded in the culture of the unit and will be sustained after the original goal has been reached
- seek and secure a commitment to provide resources on an ongoing basis.

Reflective exercise

For a practice development initiative you would like to introduce to your workplace consider the following questions:

- How is the initiative likely to be supported by key people and groups, including the nurse unit manager, nursing administration, nurse clinicians and other health professionals?

Continued

- What resources are required to implement the practice?
- Which of these resources are already available and which need to be sourced?
- How can the necessary resources that are not currently available be secured?
- What are the professional development needs of staff?
- Who are the staff members most likely to support and champion the new initiative?
- What barriers are likely to emerge as an impediment to implementing the new initiative?
- How can these barriers be overcome?
- If there is not a practice development nursing role in place, how will the momentum be obtained?
- How can the sustainability of the initiative be ensured following its implementation?

The importance of dedicated practice development roles

The commitment and enthusiasm of Jenny and other staff like her is crucial to the success of practice development initiatives. However, client care is the primary function of clinicians and the demands of contemporary health services can make it difficult to keep focused on practice development. Insufficient time is frequently cited by clinicians as a reason for not engaging in research or practice development activities. Despite Jenny's commitment, over time she may find it increasingly difficult to remain focused on the family-sensitive practice initiative, and without consistent attention the initiative is unlikely to succeed. A practice development role provides a nurse with dedicated time to ensure that momentum is not lost.

Unfortunately, not all facilities have nurses in dedicated practice development roles. The economic constraints of contemporary health care often mean that roles not directly oriented towards patient care are not well supported. Given the importance of the role it is essential that the functions of a practice development nurse are delineated and executed by one or more nurses. In the absence of a dedicated role, it is unlikely that one person will be able to fulfil all of these functions. However, it is highly desirable that one person takes responsibility for coordinating the initiative. Shared responsibility often results in busy people leaving it up to someone else or feeling too over-burdened by clinical and administrative responsibilities to find sufficient time to devote to practice development. At the end of the day one individual needs to take responsibility for assigning tasks, ensuring they are done on time and organising regular meetings.

Characteristics of practice developers

The qualities of those who lead or champion practice development initiatives are generally similar to those required for any leadership role. They need to be the type of people that others are inspired by and want to follow. Some specific qualities noted in the literature (Garbett & McCormack, 2004) include:

- enthusiasm and energy
- an optimistic view that change can happen and be sustained
- patience and the ability to recognise resistance from others without taking it too personally
- a good sense of humour
- vision – the ability to consider a better, more effective way of practicing
- empathy towards the pressures of the conditions nurses work under
- risk-taking – being prepared to try things differently even though there is no guarantee of success
- credibility – where those involved in practice development are respected by others they are more likely to create enthusiasm and to be forgiven if initiatives do not eventuate as planned.

In addition, practice developers need a broad range of skills and knowledge, including:

- creativity – in problem solving and communication
- lateral thinking
- political awareness of the ways to ensure ideas and visions are accepted both by management (who will largely control whether resources are provided) and by those at the clinical level (who will largely control whether initiatives are actually implemented at the practice level)
- good relationships with clinicians and managers
- the ability to facilitate others in the articulation, development and implementation of their ideas
- continuing a clinical role, although this is a controversial one. The need for practice developers to have a clinical load is argued primarily so that they:
  - demonstrate currency of skills
  - are seen to understand the 'real world' of clinical practice
  - become effective modellers of best practice as they work alongside other clinicians.

As mentioned above, maintaining a clinical role is controversial. Although it has the advantage of maintaining currency and credibility, given the previously discussed busyness and demands of clinical practice, the practice development nurse may feel compelled to, or succumb to pressure to, prioritise direct patient care over the practice development role.

Clinical supervision and practice development

The relationship between the two

In working through this chapter it is likely that you will already have formed ideas about the relationship between clinical supervision and practice development. If practice development aims to achieve the goal of improving the standards and quality of nursing care, in order to improve outcomes for those who use health care services, then clinical supervision must be an integral part of that development. Having said that, we are not suggesting that clinical supervision assumes responsibility for the standards and quality of nursing care, but rather it reflects our belief that the standard and quality of nursing care are likely to be enhanced by nurses who are receiving clinical supervision.

Because of their common interest in clinical practice, many would argue that in fact there is no significant difference between practice development and clinical supervision or that they are two factors in the same process. This is particularly the case for group clinical supervision (see Chapter 4). Group clinical supervision is frequently introduced as a way to encourage nurses to focus on practice issues and therefore could be the natural venue for instigating change. Stevens *et al.* (2005: 495) suggest:

> [Clinical] supervision takes a central role when changing practice as it ensures the needs of clinicians are fully supported. Monthly on-site peers supervision will provide a forum for discussing, reflecting and analysing . . . such a practice-based forum, adopting the problem-solving approach, helps dissolve any obstacles encountered by clinicians along the practice development process.

However, individual supervision can make an equally important contribution to practice development. Think back to the Hancox & Lynch (2002) definition presented in Chapter 1:

> Clinical supervision is a formal process of consultation between two or more professionals. The focus is to provide support for the supervisee(s) in order to promote self-awareness, development and growth within the context of their professional development.

The focus on self-awareness, development and growth can effectively 'set the scene' by working towards the establishment of a culture that fosters practice development. Of course the success of this strategy relies on sufficient numbers of nurses engaging in clinical supervision in order that the impact it has on the practice of individuals can be influential over the prevailing ward culture.

Refer back to Stacey's story at the beginning of this chapter. Stacey might use clinical supervision as a venue to work with her supervisor to identify ways that she could begin to have more control over her style of and approach to practice, rather than feeling she is 'putting out spot fires'. Together they might identify some techniques she could use to provide more person-centred care for her patients in spite of the barriers imposed by large workloads and staff shortages. For example, the clinical supervisor might ask Stacey questions about her practice and the difficulties she encounters. This process will increase Stacey's awareness of her work environment, both through the action of exploring the issues with someone and through this exploration being required to articulate them.

In reading Stacey's story it seems likely that she would embrace the idea of clinical supervision as a support and even see it as a possible way to enact change. Not all nurses are likely to respond so positively. The issue of whether clinical supervision should be mandatory or voluntary is an area of controversy that is discussed in Chapter 6. However, even nurses who initially refuse clinical supervision tend to notice the positive experiences of those actively engaged in it.

As Stacey and her like-minded colleagues develop a new approach to their practice, they are likely to be more satisfied and display a more positive attitude to work that can clearly be observed by others. The power of curiosity can be very strong, and the resisters may decide there might be something in this after all or at least want to find out for themselves what it is all about. From this point, hopefully their experience with clinical supervision will be a favourable one and they will become 'converted'.

It is easy to see that if enough of the nurses Stacey works with take up clinical supervision a practice development approach to their work may well become a logical next step. They will be comfortable with reflective processes and more likely to respond to change as a challenge rather than an impediment. They are likely to be more prepared to work as a team and more effective in doing so. The goals of practice development become more easily realised.

Furthermore, clinical supervision encourages nurses to take responsibility for their individual practice, which can help to avoid the tendency for practice development leaders to be seen as the 'doers' and the other nurses as the 'takers' or followers.

This is not to suggest that the need for, or importance of, clinical supervision would diminish if and when a practice development approach was introduced in the workplace. Although the needs of the team might be met through practice development, the individual needs of nurses for reflection, growth and development will continue throughout their working lives. Indeed, the health of a team depends largely on the health of its individual members. Within even the most functional teams, conflicts and specific issues will develop that a nurse may wish to examine and work through in clinical supervision.

Furthermore, teams are not static, people move on and new people enter and the broader culture of the group may change accordingly. Clinical supervision may assist nurses to view these changes as constructive rather than destructive. When change occurs people often respond initially according to the impact it has on them. In the first instance they may be aware of the loss of how things were and very anxious about how far-reaching the changes will be. The anxiety is often a mixture of the real and imagined issues they will have to face. Clinical supervision can assist people to explore the issues concerning them, helping to distinguish fantasy from reality.

Example

Becca is an associate unit manager (ANUM) who has been working for the last 12 months in very busy unit. She was encouraged to apply for the ANUM position by her nurse unit manager (NUM), whom she respects. However, the NUM has resigned and her replacement is a person Becca knows of and does not regard positively. Becca believes there will be a number of changes brought in that will be really negative. In clinical supervision Becca is asked by her supervisor to talk about the concerns she has. In doing so she comes to understand that some of her concerns are based on information from the gossip lines from some people she does not usually listen to because they are known to pass on destructive information that is not always accurate. Becca also comes to recognise that her sadness about her previous NUM leaving is also impacting on how she feels about the new NUM. She admits that she would feel somewhat disloyal to the former NUM if she likes the new NUM.

Clinical supervision is also crucial for those who assume leadership roles through the implementation of a practice development approach. Refer back to the characteristics of practice developers above. Leadership in any environment requires high levels of enthusiasm and motivation that must be maintained even in the face of resistance and opposition. Support is essential.

In addition, practice development leaders must ensure that they do not begin to become set in their ways. Leaders need to reflect on their leadership style and be willing to explore different approaches. Particularly at times when things seem to be going well, the need for self-reflection and the keen observation of ways to do things differently or better remain paramount. As the unit or team practices continue to develop and change, practice development leaders may need to develop new skills and acquire more knowledge. Clinical supervision provides the appropriate mechanism for meeting all of these ongoing needs.

We would argue therefore, that effective practice development cannot be maintained over the long term without clinical supervision. Whether this should occur individually or on a group basis will be a matter for the leadership and management groups to decide. The respective roles of individual and group supervision are considered in Chapter 4.

Reflective exercise

Think back to Vanessa, the practice development nurse, one of two nurses involved in the task of implementing change in relation to the development of family-sensitive practices on their paediatric unit. This cultural, educational and practice change requires leadership, energy and commitment, particularly in the early stages when other nurses may not yet be on board.

Clinical supervision could have a vital role in supporting and even motivating these nurses as they embark on their practice development endeavour. Just how clinical supervision and a supervisor would do this would depend on what Vanessa brought to supervision and what she wanted to use this relationship for.

For example, if Vanessa was receiving clinical supervision she might want to use a session to talk about her frustrations with the rest of the nursing team. She is very excited about the family-sensitive practice work and how it could really assist the ward but the other staff do not seem to share her passion and enthusiasm. During supervision, Vanessa tells her supervisor that she was not really aware how negative the team could be about change until this point. The only other nurse that seems keen is Jenny; after completing the course she is 'sold', but they both know that the two of them alone will not create widespread changes to practice.

Although the implementation of a family-sensitive approach is a team responsibility, Vanessa has an important role in providing support and encouragement, in keeping the team on track and in seeking the resources required. Vanessa is feeling this pressure as she feels she constantly has to drive and lead everything, that no one else is taking any responsibility.

Imagine you are Vanessa's clinical supervisor. Through supervision how would you assist Vanessa to explore her role as the leader of this new initiative? Together you could explore and review the culture of the team and begin to consider the reasons the team are resistant to the idea of family-sensitive practice. This will provide Vanessa with a safe environment to express her frustrations and concerns whilst still generating ideas and strategies on how to move forward. As a supervisor you can be a pivotal support for Vanessa while she takes on this new challenge.

Observing the differences

The fact that both clinical supervision and practice development are deeply oriented towards practice can result in confusion about the differences between the two. While the overlap is substantial, the important distinction is that clinical supervision is more closely aligned to individual professional growth and development, while practice development is more closely aligned to organisational change and the promotion of quality.

Again, look back at the Hancox and Lynch definition of clinical supervision. It clearly states that self-reflection, growth and development occur '. . . within the context of professional development'. The nurse engaged in clinical supervision may seek to explore conflict relationships, develop new skills for use in practice or work through difficulties experienced in caring for particular clients or client groups. The nurse, and his or her development as a professional, however, remains the focal point of this interaction.

In the case of practice development the focus is on changing the organisational culture in order to move towards new approaches to, or techniques of, practice. Professional development remains important within this context but it is generally directed towards the goals of organisational change rather than being ascertained by the needs and aspirations of individual nurses.

An effective and responsive organisation should view both clinical supervision and practice development as crucial for the articulation, improvement and ongoing development of nursing practice, and ultimately to achieve the highest possible standard of patient outcomes.

Conclusion

The focus of this chapter has been to highlight the similarity between the goals and purposes of practice development and clinical supervision. The ongoing development of nursing practice is central to the philosophy of both. The similarities and differences between clinical supervision and practice development have been described with emphasis on the important contribution that clinical supervision can make to practice development.

References

Commonwealth of Australia (1997) *National Mental Health Standards.* Canberra: Australian Government Publishing Service.

Commonwealth of Australia (1998) *Evaluation of the National Mental Health Strategy.* Canberra: Australian Government Publishing Service.

Commonwealth of Australia (2003) *National Mental Health Plan 2003–2008.* Canberra: Australian Government Publishing Service.

Garbett, R. & McCormack, B. (2002) A concept analysis of practice development. *Nursing Times Research*, 7(2), 87–100.

Garbett, R. & McCormack, B. (2004) A concept analysis of practice development. In: McCormack, B., Manly, K. & Garbett, R. (eds). *Practice Development in Nursing*. Oxford: Blackwell Publishing Limited, Chapter 2, pp 10–32.

Goodwin, V. & Happell, B. (2006) In our own words: consumers' views on the reality of consumer participation in mental health care. *Contemporary Nurse*, 21(1), 4–13.

Hutchinson, A.M. & Johnston, L. (2006) Beyond the BARRIERS Scale: Commonly reported barriers to research use. *Journal of Nursing Administration*, 36(4), 189–199.

Lammers, J. & Happell, B. (2004) Mental health reforms and their impact on consumer and carer participation: A perspective from Victoria, Australia. *Issues in Mental Health Nursing*, 25(3), 261–273.

McCormack, B., Manly, K. & Garbett, R. (eds) (2004) *Practice Development in Nursing*. Oxford: Blackwell Publishing Limited.

Rycroft-Malone, J. (2004) Research implementation evidence, context and facilitation – the PARIHS Framework. In: McCormack, B., Manly, K. & Garbett, R. (eds). *Practice Development in Nursing*. Oxford: Blackwell Publishing Limited, Chapter 6, pp 118–147.

Stevens, S., Sin, J., Ward, M. & Jackson, M. (2005) Practice development. Implementing a self-management model of relapse prevention for psychosis into routine clinical practice. *Journal of Psychiatric & Mental Health Nursing*, 12(4), 495–501.

Implementing clinical supervision **3**

Introduction

A structured approach to implementation has been recognised as crucial for the successful introduction of clinical supervision. As a guide to facilitate successful implementation, the aim of this chapter is to:

- introduce the importance of a structured implementation strategy
- explore the importance of organisational culture to the implementation of clinical supervision
- provide an overview of the implementation of clinical supervision within one health service
- present a research-based model designed to guide the implementation process
- explore role definition and meaning, the impact of role and the link to culture within organisations.

The importance of implementation

Despite the recent attention to clinical supervision for nursing, little consideration has been given to the implementation process. Departments of health have generally not set strong directions to assist the implementation of clinical supervision. For example, the UK Department of Health defines clinical supervision but discusses the implementation in very general terms. The initial position statement on clinical supervision for nursing and health visiting from the UK Central Council for Nursing, Midwifery and Health Visiting was scant on the detail of how to implement clinical supervision. It is argued (Mullarkey & Playle, 2001; Clifton, 2002; Riordan, 2002) that this lack of overall policy direction has contributed to difficulties in implementing clinical supervision.

Similarly in Australia, during the introduction of clinical supervision for nurses in mental health services in Victoria, scant consideration was given to the implementation process. As part of the Enterprise Bargaining Agreement of 2000, the Mental Health Branch of the Department of Human Services, Victoria, committed to funding 63 new senior nursing positions. The introduction of clinical supervision for nurses formed part of the brief of these new positions.

Despite this commitment, implementation was not addressed. Almost 6 years after the release of funding, the Clinical Supervision Guidelines in Victoria (Department of Human Services, Victoria, 2006) were finally released. This document provided a general, non-prescriptive overview for implementation. It included suggestions for policies and procedure, and recommended organisations consider an incremental implementation and make a broad reference to education and training, clinical governance and evaluation. The guidelines acknowledge different models of clinical supervision, reflecting different professional training and work contexts, and recognise that several models of clinical supervision may operate in the one organisation.

The lack of structures to guide implementation has been blamed for the failure of clinical supervision to be successfully employed as a strategy for nurses.

The importance of implementation is addressed in the work of Driscoll (2000). Successful implementation according to Driscoll begins with assessing the culture of the organisation.

Driscoll devotes a full chapter of his text to assessing the culture of the organisation. He describes the process as a journey and utilises the analogy of 'getting supervision off the ground' being the same as 'the exploits of balloonists who tried to be the first to circumnavigate the globe' (Driscoll, 2000: 158). What Driscoll means by this analogy is that just having the idea to implement clinical supervision does not make the idea work; things will not always go to plan. There may in fact be challenges along the way, such as forces at work within the culture of the organisation that either support or resist the implementation and therefore have the potential to 'blow the balloon (supervision) off course'.

Driscoll (2000: 159) describes these forces as either 'pushing or resisting forces'. Pushing forces are the strengths within the culture that assist with implementation. Resisting forces are aspects of a negative culture or a weakness that can slow down or impede implementation. As described in his text, Driscoll recommends conducting a 'force-field analysis' or an analysis of the culture of nurses/the organisation towards supervision at the beginning of the clinical supervision implementation strategy in order to identify the pushing and resisting forces, and hence assess what may be needed to assist with the implementation process.

Figure 3.1 is an adaptation from the work of Driscoll (2000) using the analogy of the balloonists. It visually represents the journey of implementation of supervision from the emerging idea to it being successfully implemented. It demonstrates the clinical supervision journey from image to action and includes the pushing and resisting forces that will affect this journey. Driscoll proposes that once the culture has been assessed and the pushing and resisting forces have been identified, the strategy then becomes strengthening and building on the pushing forces and weakening the resisting forces. For example, if there are highly motivated skilled staff in the work area (pushing force) but overall there is a lack of knowledge about clinical supervision (resisting

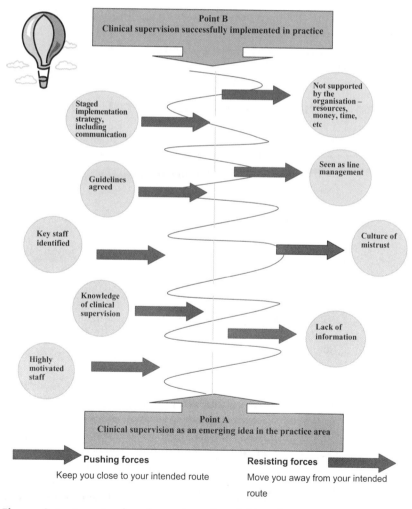

Figure 3.1   Assessing the culture using a force-field analysis.

force), then a part of the initial strategy might be coordination of motivated staff to play a large role in the initial communication strategy and promotion of clinical supervision.

Reflective exercise

Consider the organisation you work for and list:

- the pushing forces (strengthening/positive forces)
- the resisting forces(weakening/negative forces).

While other authors also refer to the importance of culture in the implementation process (Bond & Holland, 1998; Clifton, 2002), Driscoll really emphasises the need for the culture to be examined systematically and thoroughly.

Implementation in action: a practical example

As discussed in Chapter 1, in 2000 the Mental Health Branch of the Department of Human Services, Victoria, invested considerable funding in the introduction of clinical supervision for nurses through the funding of a number of senior nursing education and professional development positions. In the absence of a clear structure to guide implementation, mental health services have adopted varying approaches to introducing this new initiative.

Lynch has undertaken a study of the implementation journey for one Victorian mental health service (Lynch & Happell, 2008a–c). The findings from this research have led to the development of a new model for implementation. An overview of the research methods and findings are presented here, followed by a description of the model and how it can effectively be used as an instrument for the successful implementation of clinical supervision.

Study setting

The study was conducted in a large rural mental health service in south-east Victoria providing a range of mental health services to over 3000 registered clients aged 0–65+. The service covered over 44 000 km^2 and consisted of eight community centres and two inpatient units. Approximately 200 mental health clinicians were employed, 144 of whom were nurses. This service was chosen primarily because a considered implementation strategy was clearly evident. Also, it was felt that the rural organisation faced particular challenges when implementing clinical supervision, including:

- the distance required to travel for supervision
- the dual relationships within the service and the overall closeness of rural communities
- the limited number of clinical supervisor options available as cross-service clinical supervision was seen to be difficult to implement because of the tyranny of distance.

It was therefore thought that potential barriers and complexities were more likely to occur with implementation in a rural setting.

Design

The study involved three forms of data collection: an audit of all documentation pertaining to clinical supervision within the organisation, including minutes of meetings and a copy of the organisation's strategic/business plan for implementing clinical supervision; individual interviews with senior nurses and members of the implementation committee; and focus groups with nurses currently providing (supervisors) and receiving (supervisees) supervision.

The documentation was analysed using the 'force-field analysis' approach described by Driscoll (2000). Secondly, the action plan was formulated, which included looking for how, and if, the organisation strengthened and built on the pushing forces and minimised the impact of the resisting forces. The findings from this task helped to formulate the questions for the individual interviews; they formed the basis for questions pertaining to culture, implementation and the experiences of implementation.

The findings suggested that the implementation process occurred in five stages, as represented in Table 3.1.

Table 3.1 Implementation process – stages and influencing factors.

Stages	Influencing factors
Exploration	Organisational culture Exploring the possibilities
The initial implementation strategy	Leadership Organisational culture Education and training The project/strategic plan
The strategic plan	Reflection Clinical supervision implementation committee The strategic plan
Implementing the strategic plan	Clinical supervision committee Education and training Organisational culture
Reflecting on the past and moving forward	Organisational culture – culture change Sustainability On reflection

Stage 1: Exploration

This first stage was a process of exploration, which involved assessing the culture of the mental health service and determining the supports available to overcome barriers and support implementation. The influencing factors were found to be:

- organisational culture
- exploring the possibilities.

Organisational culture

A review of the organisational culture identified poor morale and a perception by staff that they were not supported by the organisation. Consequently, many had developed a distrust of management, as evidenced by high levels of nursing burnout and dissatisfaction with the work environment. A negative culture is certainly not unique to this organisation. However, once this culture was identified and named via staff satisfaction and climate surveys, senior management took a very brave step and, rather than keeping their heads in the sand, they began to discuss this negativity openly and honestly to explore what could be done to address these concerns.

Exploring the possibilities

Senior management recognised that something needed to be done to improve morale but were not sure what or how. The team began to explore options such as educational support, staff support, structural and system changes, and the need to find a new solution as described in the following statement:

> A number of senior nurses and managers had prior experience with clinical supervision personally and they felt quite strongly about the potential benefits for nurses based on their own experiences. Following initial discussions at a senior management level, an in-principle decision was made to explore the implementation of clinical supervision. Discussions had been held with a senior nurse in another organisation about the value of clinical supervision and the idea of an education program being offered. A decision was then made to formally collaborate with this other organisation.

Stage 2: The initial implementation strategy

Once the decision had been made to support the introduction of clinical supervision, attention was directed towards strategies for making this happen. The influencing factors at this point in time were identified as:

- leadership
- organisational culture
- education and training.

Leadership

A considerable amount of thought and energy went into finding the 'right leader' and 'right leadership group' to lead the change. Identifying clinical 'champions' to lead the implementation of clinical supervision has been recognised as an important strategy in other implementation programs. Clifton (2002) suggests:

> ...a champion is needed to ensure the continuing leadership for the project. The absence of someone to steer or lead the process of implementation at team and organisational level often means that progress slows down. (p. 37)

Organisational culture

Once the initial leadership group was established the committee again focused on the organisational culture. The anti-management feeling continued to be apparent. Nurses tended to be cynical and pessimistic about anything senior management tried to implement and they had little or no faith in their ability to 'sustain anything'. The staff expressed concern that clinical supervision was just the new 'in' thing and would disappear in a month or so, just like everything else that was implemented.

However, the financial commitment shown by the organisation and the early decision to collaborate with other organisations enhanced the credibility of the initiative.

Education and training

An external provider was contracted by the organisation and the collaborating service to tailor an education and training package to their needs. External training was chosen because it encouraged networking outside the organisation, reflected an independent approach, and avoided the perception that clinical supervision would be management driven. This decision was supported by the implementation team, the supervisors and the supervisees, although some participants considered a combination between internal and external facilitators may have combined independence with knowledge of the local context and culture.

Participants in the first course stated clearly that it was a huge success as it clarified for them the various types of clinical supervision and what it could offer. It provided valuable information on the legal and ethical considerations to be taken into account, the models of supervision and also presented overall information on how to implement clinical supervision for the individual/organisation.

As part of the formal assessment for the 4-day course, the participants completed a strategic plan as a group project. This was seen as a very useful basis for continuing the implementation process.

Stage 3: The strategic plan

This stage involved the finalisation and formalisation of the strategic plan and included the following influencing factors:

* reflection
* the clinical supervision implementation committee
* the strategic plan.

Reflection

After completing the first training program, the leadership group reviewed their progress thus far. They felt confident they were on track and had achieved their initial goals of obtaining organisational support, formalising the collaboration with another organisation, identifying a clearly defined leader and other key members of staff, and engaging the external provider to provide training and education. The next goal focused on the task of completing the strategic plan.

Clinical supervision implementation committee

A committee was formed to complete the strategic plan. It did not have a formal structure, although each member had defined roles and responsibilities. The committee divided tasks into those that were completed by the whole group and individual or smaller group tasks. Tasks completed by the whole group included writing the project background and overview, the vision values and mission statement, the project's aims and objectives, information about the implementation strategy and an information package including articles on models, examples of clinical supervision agreements, record forms and other references articles. Individuals or smaller groups took responsibility for marketing, policy writing and evaluation. Members of the committee appeared to self-select into tasks they were interested in or felt they had the skills to contribute to.

This self-selection of role and the lack of a formal committee structure led to some difficulties within the group, largely due to different approaches and styles and the lack of recognised leadership and a formal decision-making process. However, despite difficulties the project was completed and presented to the senior management team of the organisation.

The strategic plan

The strategic plan included the following information:

- project overview
- mission statement reflecting the values and mission of the organisation
- aims of clinical supervision
- background and current status of clinical supervision within the organisation
- definition of clinical supervision
- models of clinical supervision that could be offered
- policy and procedures
- documentation, including example agreements, record forms and references.

The tasks completed by individual or smaller groups included:

- communication and marketing
- policy and procedures
- evaluation.

Communication and marketing

The first step involved choosing a theme. This theme (growing together) formed the central part of all the material developed to promote clinical supervision. This material consisted of a clinical supervision information folder, a poster and an official launch. Figure 3.2 is the poster developed for this purpose. The poster raised awareness and provided a focus for clinical supervision activity.

The philosophy behind all aspects of the marketing strategy was to ensure that the same information was communicated to everyone to demonstrate that management was supporting the implementation and to ensure that myths and misconceptions were addressed.

An official launch of clinical supervision was held at a central location and was opened by senior management. Invitations to the launch were personally sent to all staff and due to the geographical distances teleconferencing to all sites was arranged. At the local sites the marketing committee organised a member of the clinical supervision implementation committee to welcome staff and be available for questions, arranged afternoon tea, balloons and decorations, and made sure a copy of the information folder and posters were kept at the local sites. The launch was seen as a successful marketing strategy, although participants acknowledged it was difficult to convince staff to attend.

Policies and procedures

Having clearly defined policies and protocols was seen as an important component of implementation. The original protocol was written in

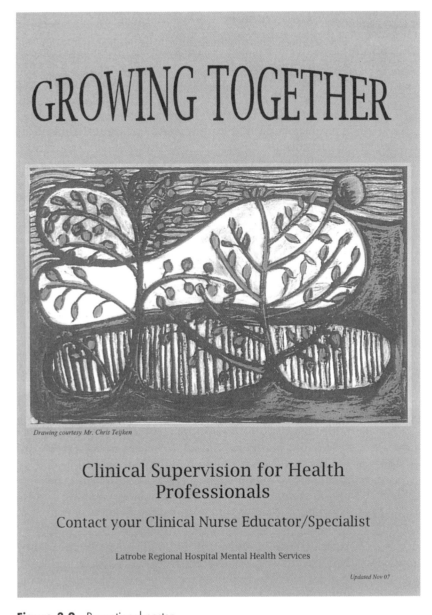

Figure 3.2 Promotional poster.

draft form and was subsequently refined following feedback from the broader staff group.

Evaluation
Evaluation was also considered essential and the organisation participated in both internal and external evaluation. The internal evaluation

was coordinated by two committee members as their primary portfolio.

Stage 4: Implementing the strategic plan

The fourth stage of the implementation strategy focused on actually implementing the strategic plan and moving to the next phase. The influencing factors identified during this stage included:

- the clinical supervision committee
- education and training
- organisational culture and support.

Clinical supervision committee

The implementation committee became more formalised and was renamed the Clinical Supervision Working Party. Membership was opened to other interested parties, such as senior nurses, nurse managers and nurses with experience in clinical supervision. The clinical supervision portfolio holder chaired the meetings and they adhered to the formal meeting structure of the organisation. There was a general discussion on topics, which were formulated into agreed actions, and people were assigned to each of the actions and deadlines were identified. The participants interviewed noted this change of structure in a positive way; there was now clarity and a clearly defined leader in the group. Participants found this structure reassuring and it appeared to address some of the concerns expressed previously in relation to the lack of a defined committee structure.

Education and training

Education and training again formed a large part of the fourth phase of the implementation strategy. Further training was contracted via the external facilitators to ensure enough staff were available to provide supervision. It was felt that some managers had little or no idea about clinical supervision and that although they were supportive, training and education were required for them to understand the concept and dispel any myths. The second group therefore was mainly senior and program managers.

Organisational culture

The inclusion of senior managers in the training program met with a mixed reaction. On the positive side it demonstrated management commitment (particularly as managers attended the course in their own time). On the negative side it reinforced some of the paranoia that clinical supervision would be controlled by management.

As a response to this feedback the clinical supervision committee decided on a nomination process to decide the participants in future courses. The committee wrote a personal letter to everyone who had attended the 1-day workshop (Introduction to supervision) and asked them all to nominate five people they would access for clinical supervision if they had a choice. The results were collated by the clinical supervision portfolio holder. The people most frequently nominated were informed that they had been nominated by their peers and their interest in the training was sought. This was seen as a very creative and innovative strategy by the members of the clinical supervision working party, and it was credited with changing some of the perceptions within the organisation about the relationship between clinical supervision and line management.

Stage 5: Reflecting on the past and moving forward

The final stage focused on reflecting on the past and looking towards the future. The influencing factors included:

- organisational culture
- sustainability
- in hindsight.

Organisational culture

The participants reflected on the culture of the organisation as a way of evaluating the successful implementation strategy. The participants expressed excitement and enthusiasm about what they perceived as an enormous change of culture within the mental health program. They felt strongly that clinical supervision had been instrumental in this change. The estimated 80% of people initially negative and suspicious about clinical supervision was now judged to be only 15–30%.

Sustainability

The participants in the supervisor and supervisee focus groups identified that the fact that clinical supervision was still available 2 or 3 years after the initial idea proved to them it was sustainable. That in itself was identified as a major improvement for this organisation. Despite this confidence in the overall implementation and the success thus far, there was still some fear or apprehension expressed that clinical supervision would not be sustained in the long term.

Initial evaluation findings suggest that the implementation of clinical supervision was successful. The need for ongoing research, evaluation and quality assurance activities was identified and plans were made to conduct research and evaluation in the future to assist with the sustainability and continue to monitor the successes and challenges. Given the considerable financial costs of implementing clinical supervision, favourable outcomes need to be demonstrated to ensure that the support continues. It was estimated that the cost of wages alone based on one session per nurse every 3 weeks would equate to $10000 per month.

Sustainability has involved working with senior managers on service mapping to review other structural and management processes so that any budget cuts would not threaten the viability of clinical supervision.

Other challenges of sustainability include maintaining the motivation and enthusiasm of the working group and all nursing staff, outgrowing supervisors and accessing all nurses within the mental health program. There was a definite consensus in all of the findings that nursing staff felt that clinical supervision was still vulnerable to the implementation faltering or the process being replaced by something new.

On reflection

The participants described what they had learnt from the process, and what they would change. One participant reflected on the feelings of accountability in the initial part of the implementation process, the responsibilities of being a leader. However, this participant and others felt that this had changed and now there was joint responsibility and motivation for the sustainability of clinical supervision. In hindsight, this participant suggested that perhaps there should have been two leaders or 'champions' formally identified for a project of this magnitude.

Supervisees identified that during the initial phase of introducing clinical supervision a survey could have been circulated in order to gain an understanding of what the knowledge base was in relation to clinical supervision throughout the organisation. The communication and marketing strategy could have therefore been even more 'tailored to meet the specific organisational needs'. The survey results could have also been used to demonstrate the changes in the organisation and compare the findings with other organisations seeking to implement clinical supervision.

In relation to the education and training strategy, a couple of participants continued to express their concern about managers completing the 4-day training and even recommended a modified training course for the management team that just emphasised what clinical supervision was and how it could best be implemented. This ongoing concern from staff, however, suggests that the importance of involving managers in order to gain their support was not clearly conveyed or appreciated.

Other suggestions of implementation strategies that participants would change in hindsight included asking for expressions of interest in being a clinical supervisor as well as the nominations, making sure there was an even spread of clinical supervisors trained throughout the region, ensuring there were enough staff trained and ready prior to the launch and lobbying for funding specifically for research.

Summary of research findings

The implementation of clinical supervision occurred across five stages:

- the initial exploration of what the organisation needed
- the forming of ideas on how clinical supervision could be implemented
- the formulation of the strategic plan
- operationalising the strategic plan
- the process of reflection and evaluation.

In each of these stages, a number of influencing factors emerged, some of which appeared in a number of stages.

A model for the implementation of clinical supervision

As stated previously, a force-field analysis, based on the work of Driscoll (2000), was conducted following the documentation audit to identify the forces that might facilitate the implementation of this new initiative and those that might detract from it. The force-field analysis is presented in Figure 3.3.

Driscoll's model provided a simple and structured way to analyse the documentation and gain a baseline understanding of the organisation's preparedness. However, two significant limitations became apparent:

- The importance of one strategy over another is not identified with this approach. Forces are identified as positive or negative, not how influential these forces are.
- The underlying assumption is that the assessment of organisational culture takes place prior to the implementation process. This does not reflect the dynamic nature of organisations and the continual competition for scarce financial resources.

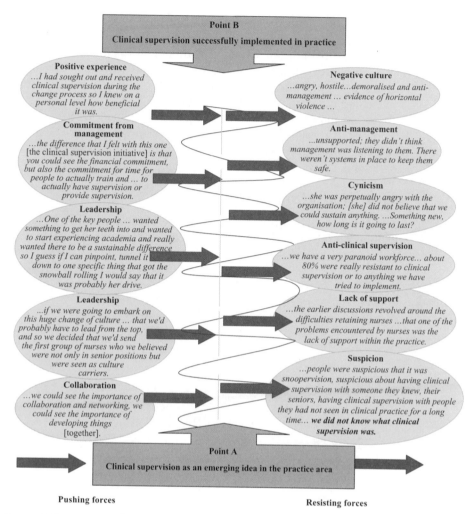

Positive experience
...I had sought out and received clinical supervision during the change process so I knew on a personal level how beneficial it was.

Negative culture
...angry, hostile...demoralised and anti-management ... evidence of horizontal violence ...

Commitment from management
...the difference that I felt with this one [the clinical supervision initiative] is that you could see the financial commitment, but also the commitment for time for people to actually train and ... to actually have supervision or provide supervision.

Anti-management
...unsupported; they didn't think management was listening to them. There weren't systems in place to keep them safe.

Leadership
...One of the key people ... wanted something to get her teeth into and wanted to start experiencing academia and really wanted there to be a sustainable difference so I guess if I can pinpoint, tunnel it down to one specific thing that got the snowball rolling I would say that it was probably her drive.

Cynicism
...she was perpetually angry with the organisation; [she] did not believe that we could sustain anything. ...Something new, how long is it going to last?

Anti-clinical supervision
...we have a very paranoid workforce... about 80% were really resistant to clinical supervision or to anything we have tried to implement.

Leadership
...if we were going to embark on this huge change of culture ... that we'd probably have to lead from the top, and so we decided that we'd send the first group of nurses who we believed were not only in senior positions but were seen as culture carriers.

Lack of support
...the earlier discussions revolved around the difficulties retaining nurses ...that one of the problems encountered by nurses was the lack of support within the practice.

Collaboration
...we could see the importance of collaboration and networking, we could see the importance of developing things [together].

Suspicion
*...people were suspicious that it was snoopervision, suspicious about having clinical supervision with someone they knew, their seniors, having clinical supervision with people they had not seen in clinical practice for a long time... **we did not know what clinical supervision was.***

Point B
Clinical supervision successfully implemented in practice

Point A
Clinical supervision as an emerging idea in the practice area

Pushing forces

Resisting forces

Figure 3.3   Assessing the culture and preparedness to implement clinical supervision.

Reflective exercise

Earlier in the chapter you were asked to assess the culture of your organisation and record the pushing and resisting forces. Refer back to that list and consider the following questions:

- Do you consider all of the identified forces to be of equal impact?
- If not, rate each of them as strong, medium or weak.
- For both pushing and resisting forces add up the number in each category.
- Assess which emerges as having the stronger impact: pushing or resisting.

These limitations and the research findings led to the development of the Lynch model to guide implementation, reflecting the dynamic and changing nature of organisations. The model allows for the assessment of the impact or influence of the pushing and resisting forces, and encourages regular and ongoing assessments of the culture. This model is presented diagrammatically in Figure 3.4.

There are many key discussions, decisions and actions that need to be completed at each step before being able to move on to the next step. Overall details about each step, including the primary key tasks, are described below.

Step 1: Clinical supervision or . . . ?

At this stage a decision needs to be made about a number of factors surrounding the essential initial question – Why clinical supervision?

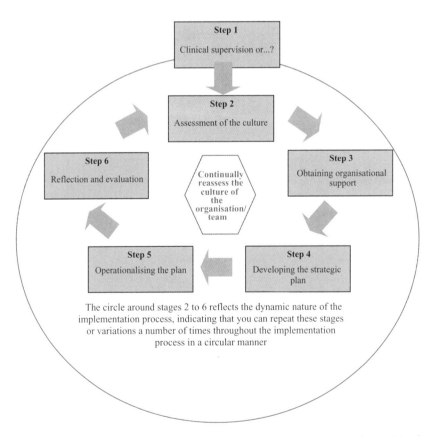

Figure 3.4 Clinical supervision for your organisation – the Lynch model of implementation.

(1) What does the organisation want for its nurses/employees?
(2) Why is clinical supervision being considered?
(3) What is the organisation really looking for? Is it really clinical supervision or has the organisation confused the concept of clinical supervision with some of the commonly confused other forums/concepts (see Chapter 1)? Is the organisation really talking about another concept entirely, such as management supervision, mentorship, preceptorship or performance management?
(4) What will clinical supervision look like? In other words, how is clinical supervision to be defined and how will it interface with the existing structures and disciplines other than nursing?
(5) How will clinical supervision be offered? What is the overall goal of implementation, e.g. implement individual/group or a combination of both?

The implementation of clinical supervision for nurses is a complex and challenging task; it takes time, energy, dedication and commitment. It is at this first stage that a decision needs to be made about whether it is worth embarking on this journey.

Key tasks

(1) Establish leadership and identify key staff to drive the implementation. These people will be the key drivers of the implementation through to steps 4 and 5 when there are more opportunities for other interested clinicians to join an implementation committee or working party.
(2) Consult three or four of these people on the following questions:
- Ask yourselves the questions in step 1 of the model to explore whether you and your organisation wants clinical supervision or something else entirely.
- Do you think clinical supervision would be beneficial to the organisation?
- Do you think clinical supervision could be successfully implemented within the organisation?

Step 2: Assessment of the culture

Understanding the culture of the organisation is essential. Completing the initial assessment (force-field analysis) of the culture provides a baseline in order to determine the organisation's preparedness and also provides a direction for the next steps in the implementation strategy.

Key tasks

(1) Conduct a force-field analysis to clearly identify the pushing and resisting forces. This can be represented diagrammatically or written as a list (Driscoll, 2000). Surveys may need to be conducted in order to accurately assess the pushing or resisting forces. Again this initial survey may also be useful in establishing the baseline knowledge of clinical supervision and the extent to which staff are interested in pursuing clinical supervision (supervisor/supervisee roles).

(2) Discuss these findings to determine how important each of these pushing and resisting forces are. Ultimately, this will be based on the organisation's subjective views and opinions.

(3) With this priority list in mind the next step is to develop an action plan that will identify how you plan to address the pushing and resisting forces. This plan should be listed in order of importance and level of influence. In addition, it is important to identify the roles and responsibilities that individuals have within the initial action plan (Bond & Holland, 1998).

Table 3.2 provides an example of an action plan. You may like to use this one or design your own. Remember it needs to include the task, whether it is a pushing or a resisting force, the actions needed to address the force and finally ensure that those responsible are named with a time frame/review date clearly articulated.

Step 3: Obtaining organisational support

Gaining organisational support is essential and requires recognition as a step in the implementation model. The information collected in steps 1 and 2 assists in identifying what organisational support is needed. Step 3 therefore confirms this need and ensures that the organisation will provide the necessary resources before time and energy are used moving to the next stage.

Table 3.2 Action plan: the next steps – priorities and responsibilities.

Task (in order of importance)	Pushing/ resisting force	Action plan to address the force	Person(s) responsible	Time frame
Vision and leadership	Pushing	'Vision, courage, creativity, effective communication and a clear plan' (Daly *et al.*, 2004: 185).	Leader and implementation team	
Anti-management negative culture and lack of knowledge	Resisting	Leadership and vision and an education and training strategy – using external facilitators	Leader and team and the external educators	

Reflective exercise

- Brainstorm what resources you think you need to implement clinical super-vision (remember the force-field analysis should give you the information you need to ascertain what resources you might need).
- List these resources in order of importance – again this is influenced by your assessment of the organisational culture.
- Identify and list the key people in your organisation who could help you with the resources you need.

The following example demonstrates the possible stages involved in determining the level of organisational support needed in relation to providing education and training. This process reinforces that the support needed from the organisation can differ, as it is dependent on the findings from steps 1 and 2. Figure 3.5 articulates an example of how this can occur.

Once organisational support has been secured, leadership and con-sultation become crucial for the coordination and writing of the strate-gic plan. This plan should include consultation by conducting surveys or face-to-face via individual interviews, focus groups and/or public forums with key stakeholders. Some of the key stakeholders relevant to the implementation of clinical supervision for nurses are:

- department/organisation executive
- nurse educators
- nurse managers
- external trainers or facilitators
- clinically based nurses of varying levels
- other collaborating agencies and key stakeholders in the organisation.

Key tasks

(1) List the key stakeholders within your organisation.
(2) Briefly develop a consultation plan, i.e. how should these people or groups be accessed? Whose support do you need (for example, the support of the unit manager would be crucial in accessing ward staff)?
(3) Develop a communication strategy to ensure that clear and accurate infor-mation is provided to all staff (to minimise the potential impact of myths and misconceptions).
(4) Draft a timeline for consultation.
(5) Identify what resources will be needed at this stage, e.g. time release, other staff to assist with consultation, administrative support.
(6) Identify how these resources can be obtained.

Step 1: Decision regarding implementing clinical supervision for nurses

Step 2: Assessment of the culture, e.g. force-field analysis focusing on knowledge of clinical supervision

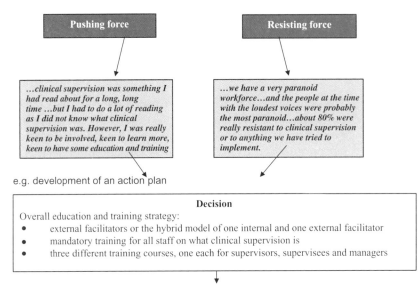

Pushing force

Resisting force

...clinical supervision was something I had read about for a long, long time ...but I had to do a lot of reading as I did not know what clinical supervision was. However, I was really keen to be involved, keen to learn more, keen to have some education and training

...we have a very paranoid workforce...and the people at the time with the loudest voices were probably the most paranoid...about 80% were really resistant to clinical supervision or to anything we have tried to implement.

e.g. development of an action plan

Decision

Overall education and training strategy:
- external facilitators or the hybrid model of one internal and one external facilitator
- mandatory training for all staff on what clinical supervision is
- three different training courses, one each for supervisors, supervisees and managers

Step 3: Gaining organisational support

Organisational support required

Given the level of mistrust, paranoia and the lack of knowledge about clinical supervision at all levels of the organisation, commitment was needed from the organisation to provide resources for external facilitators. The main resource would include funding for the training, including accommodation and backfill.

Figure 3.5 Obtaining organisational support.

The views and opinions expressed during the consultation process should inform the overall development of the plan. The actual strategic plan should include:

- introduction and overview: the vision, mission and the overall aims and objectives for the implementation of clinical supervision
- background and information regarding the rationale for the intro-duction of clinical supervision (collected during the consultation phase)
- definition of clinical supervision
- implementation strategy – the action plan that identifies tasks, roles and timelines

- education and training strategy
- communication and marketing strategy
- policies and protocols
- evaluation/research
- all documentation, including copies of agreements, record forms and references
- any other issues considered important that reflect the specific context or needs of the individual organisation.

Step 4: Developing the strategic plan

Once organisational support has been secured, this is the stage where the leaders and other chosen key nurses need to do an enormous amount of work to coordinate and write the strategic plan. This plan should include consultation by conducting surveys or face-to-face individual interviews, or using focus groups and/or public forums with key stakeholders. Examples of some of the key stakeholders relevant to the implementation of clinical supervision for nurses are:

- department executive
- nurse educators
- nurse managers
- external trainers/facilitators
- representation of the nurses in the organisation
- other collaborating agencies and key stakeholders in the organisation.

The views and opinions expressed during the consultation process should inform the overall development of the plan. The actual strategic plan then needs to be developed. According to the findings from this research, supported by the literature, the strategic plan should at a minimum include:

- introduction and overview: the vision, mission and overall aims and objectives for the implementation of clinical supervision
- background and information pertaining to why clinical supervision (information collected in step 1)
- definition of clinical supervision
- implementation strategy in detail (this may include the analysis of the culture or the action plan that identifies tasks, roles and timelines)
- education and training strategy
- communication and marketing strategy
- policies and protocols
- evaluation/research
- all documentation, including copies of agreements, record forms and references.

Step 5: Operationalising the plan

This involves formalising a clinical supervision committee/working party and operationalising the strategic plan. The main parts of the plan that will be the most active in this step are the education and training, and the communication/marketing strategy.

Key tasks

(1) Identify potential members for the implementation committee.
(2) Ensure that membership reflects:
   • people with interest, passion and motivation
   • people with the capacity to influence resource allocation
   • people respected across the organisation
   • people representing a range of positions and experience
   • people with expertise in a range of areas including:
      ○ education and training
      ○ communication and marketing
      ○ research and evaluation
(3) Consider how you would structure the meeting to ensure maximum attendance.
(4) Organise someone to distribute agendas and take minutes.

Education and training

The education and training strategy chosen must be compatible with the organisation. Figure 3.6 provides a summary of some of the factors that should be considered in selecting the most appropriate option.

Communication and marketing

Communication and marketing are essential to 'sell' clinical supervision to nurses. The findings from step 2 will suggest how aggressive the marketing strategy needs to be and the findings from step 3 will indicate what resources are available for this part of the strategy.

Developing an action plan/tracking score card at this stage may be useful to ensure that all parts of the strategic plan are operationalised. An example of a tracking scorecard that could be used for this purpose is provided in Table 3.3.

Reflective exercise

Using the blank tracking scorecard in Table 3.4 list important activities that need to be achieved, the person(s) responsible and information regarding time frames.

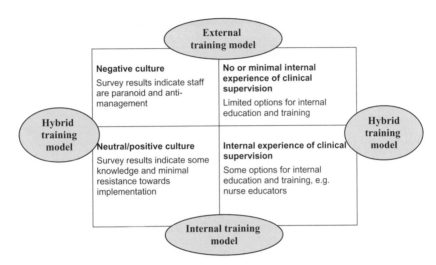

Figure 3.6   Choosing the type of education and training required.

Table 3.3   Tracking score card – a communication tool.

Activity — Monthly review	Person(s) responsible	Reviewed monthly					
		Jan	Feb	March	April	May	June
Design survey to assess staff knowledge of clinical supervision	Project lead	1	2	X			
Decide the most effective way to implement the survey	Project lead		1	1	X	2	
Collate findings of the survey	Project lead and nurse with research experience					1	1
Complete the force-field analysis	Project lead executive sponsor		1	1	1	2	X
Obtain organisational support (in writing)	Executive sponsor	3	3	3	3	X	

1, commenced; 2, completed; 3, behind schedule; X, due.

Table 3.4 Tracking score card – a communication tool (blank).

Activity (in order of priority)	Person(s) responsible	Reviewed monthly					
Monthly review		Jan	Feb	March	April	May	June

1, commenced; 2, completed; 3, behind schedule; X, due.

Step 6: Reflection and evaluation

The final stage is about reflection and evaluation of the strategy thus far and an opportunity to consider issues of sustainability in the future of clinical supervision within the organisation.

It is necessary to reassess the culture of the organisation (as in step 2) to determine the current climate. An evaluation process should be implemented to assess the success of the project according to the original aims and objectives. If the results suggest the aims and objectives have not been met, the clinical supervision implementation committee may need to revisit the model and repeat a variation of steps 3, 4 and 5.

For example, if the findings show that there are still a number of staff members who do not understand clinical supervision, the committee may need to renegotiate with the organisation for additional resources for education, training and marketing.

At this stage issues of sustainability need to be discussed and some of the future plans may involve publications, conference presentations, additional research and a review of the strategic plan to see what additional resources (e.g. new training programs) are available or to reflect changes in service structure that may have implications for initiatives such as clinical supervision.

And so the circle continues . . .

The model presented in Figure 3.4 has a circle around steps 2 to 6. This reflects the dynamic nature of the implementation process. It represents flexibility in allowing for constant revision and reassessment where the implementation process is not completely successful immediately. Even when successful implementation has occurred it is likely that broader organisational and political changes will require modifications. The reassessment process provides the foundations to continually assess the culture of the organisation to sense what the current climate is. Organisational culture has an enormous impact on the success/failure of both the initial implementation and its sustainability.

Conclusion

There is sufficient evidence to suggest that clinical supervision could be an important strategy in overcoming problems with retention of the nursing workforce. A considered and structured plan for the implementation of clinical supervision is crucial to the success of this strategy. Indeed, an ad hoc, disorganised and uncoordinated way of introducing clinical supervision could actually reinforce the surrounding common myths and paranoia, and significantly reduce the potential positive benefits. Despite this, most state and territory governments in Australia have consistently failed to introduce guidelines to effectively assist with the implementation process. Clinical supervision can be successfully implemented, providing a structured and systematic approach is followed. A model for implementation has been presented in this chapter. It is important to remember that the implementation of clinical supervision is an ongoing and dynamic process; continual assessment of the culture (including the recognition of pushing and resisting forces) is required.

References

Bond, M. & Holland, S. (1998) *Skills of Supervision for Nurses*. Oxford: Open University Press.

Clifton, E. (2002) Implementing clinical supervision. *Nursing Times*, 98(9), 36–37.

Daly, J., Speedy, S. & Jackson, D. (2004) *Nursing Leadership*. Marrickville, NSW: Elsevier.

Department of Human Services, Victoria (2006) Guidelines for clinical supervision. Melbourne: Department of Human Services. www.dhs.vic.gov.au/mentalhealth.

Driscoll, J. (2000) *Practicing Clinical Supervision: A Reflective Approach*. London: Balliere Tindall.

Lynch, L. & Happell, B. (2008a) Implementing clinical supervision. Part 1: Laying the ground work. *International Journal of Mental Health Nursing*, 17(1), 57–64.

Lynch, L. & Happell, B. (2008b) Implementing clinical supervision. Part 2: Implementation and beyond. *International Journal of Mental Health Nursing*, 17(1), 65–72.

Lynch, L. & Happell, B. (2008c) Implementing clinical supervision. Part 3: The development of a model. *International Journal of Mental Health Nursing*, 17(1), 73–82.

Mullarkey, K. & Playle, J. (2001) Multi professional clinical supervision: Challenges for mental health nurses. *Journal of Psychiatric and Mental Health Nursing*, 8, 205–211.

Riordan, B. (2002) Why nurses choose not to undertake CS: The findings from one ICU. *Nursing in Critical Care*, 7(2), 59–66.

Approaches to clinical supervision 4

Introduction

The aim of this chapter is to:

- distinguish between individual and group clinical supervision
- consider the implications for the use of individual vs group clinical supervision
- consider the advantages and disadvantages of external and internal clinical supervision
- discuss the relative advantages and disadvantages of multi-disciplinary vs discipline-specific clinical supervision.

Clinical supervision: individual or group?

There are specific advantages and disadvantages to individual and group clinical supervision. One is not better than the other. However, as different processes they meet different needs and purposes. Unfortunately, the decision is often economically driven, with group supervision sometimes chosen because the one facilitator can get the job done with a number of staff at the same time. This is particularly the case for nursing, where the large numbers make the job of providing supervision appear quite daunting.

Saving money or improving efficiencies should not be the primary indicator for group supervision. Group supervision is indeed about providing supervision to a group rather than a number of individuals who happen to be situated together. Group supervision should be primarily oriented towards working with a team or unit to explore the team dynamics, improve clinical skills or enhance professional development, rather than addressing the specific needs of the individuals present, that is the focus is on the collective rather than its component parts.

So what approach are you and/or your organisation considering? The following questions can assist you in making an informed decision about the best approach to take.

Is the goal to work with the individual nurse's needs and development?

If the answer is yes, then individual supervision will be more suitable. The group setting will not provide sufficient time for attention to be focused on the specific needs of individuals.

Is team functioning and dynamics of greatest importance?

If yes, then group supervision would be the most suitable approach as the aim of group supervision is to work with teams, and team functioning can be effectively dealt with by this approach, rather than through each team member having individual clinical supervision (although this may still be required for different reasons).

Will people feel comfortable having clinical supervision in a group setting?

The level of comfort and the ability for team members to feel they can be open and honest is crucial if group supervision is to work effectively. No matter what the potential value of the group setting, if there is no trust and members do not feel able to communicate openly, group supervision will not achieve its potential and will be more likely to have a damaging effect.

What are the skills of the clinical supervisor? Is she or he comfortable and experienced working with individuals and/or groups?

Individual and group supervision require different skills, and there is no reason to assume that a person skilled in providing individual supervision will necessarily have the confidence and competence to be able to perform in a group situation and vice versa. A supervisor who is inexperienced in this setting is likely to have difficulty in keeping the group focused or dealing with any conflict that may arise. If the supervisor is inexperienced the effects could be disastrous rather than just ineffective. It is likely to have strong negative implications that may deter the participants from any involvement in clinical supervision in the future.

What is the motivation for clinical supervision now? Has there been an event or something significant that has been the catalyst?

Sometimes the decision to engage in supervision follows a specific event or incident within the team. For example:

- The team leader or unit manager may leave and the team may feel the need for help to regroup in order to move forward with new leadership.
- An unforeseen event may occur, for example a patient dies unexpectedly as the result of complications of treatment or surgery.

If there has been a catalyst what are people hoping will be achieved through clinical supervision?

It is important that participants have a realistic view of what clinical supervision can achieve. In the first example above it might provide the opportunity for staff to reflect, to imagine their preferred future. A change in leadership can be a time of challenge and/or opportunity. A process which enables group members to reflect and consider can assist them to move forward productively, where they might otherwise flounder. Exploring these issues would be a reasonable expectation of group supervision. On the other hand, if group members were hoping that the clinical supervisor would provide advice and guidance to help them move forward, this would appear more like facilitating a strategic planning session and would not be a reasonable expectation of clinical supervision.

   In the case of the second example, group clinical supervision might be used to assist the team to come to terms with the incident, and to learn from the experience in order that, where possible, they might avoid a similar incident in the future. However, it is important to note that clinical supervision is not a reactive process following a critical incident and should not be used in this way. Following a critical incident, debriefing via an experienced clinician trained in briefing procedures should be offered to all staff involved in the incident.

Example

David is a 22-year-old single man diagnosed with bowel cancer. He is due to have surgery the next day. David has previously been treated for depression by his GP. He states that he is not coping well with the thought of having a colostomy. He has not told his girlfriend because he feels this would be 'the end of our relationship'. On admission he is quiet but communicates well when approached. He states he is feeling a bit better and is coming to terms with the

Continued

surgery but still does not want to tell his girlfriend about the colostomy, saying 'How would you feel if you had shit coming out of your belly?'. David's parents and two siblings are very supportive and caring. Later that afternoon David is found to be missing. At first the staff assume he has gone for a walk around the hospital. It is a busy shift and 2 hours pass before the staff become concerned about David's whereabouts. Attempts are made to contact his family but they are on their way in to see him. After they find out that David is missing they begin a search. After some time David is found dead in the garage of a school friend.

Whilst debriefing was provided following David's death, the unit staff wanted to explore the issues further through supervision. This would not be a suitable time to commence group clinical supervision. Indeed, this approach would really only be possible when supervision is already an established part of the team and the supervisor is known to the staff. It is not an appropriate time to commence clinical supervision following an event such as this. However, where clinical supervision is established, staff may use group clinical supervision to:

- express their grief and distress at what has occurred
- discuss how this has impacted on them as individuals and as part of the team in terms of their professional esteem
- develop a realistic view of the situation, for example the supervisor might challenge statements like: 'I/we should have known this would happen', with statements like 'How could you have known this would happen?'
- encourage the team to explore whether there were any clues that were missed and was there anything that they would pay more attention to in the future?

It is not the clinical supervisor's role to review the incident in detail, searching for errors or where to assign blame. The supervisor's role is purely to assist staff to reflect and explore the incident, particularly in relation to the thoughts and feelings of the team, and the impact that David's death has had on them. If the supervisor was using a reflective model of clinical supervision he or she may also reflect on the incident and strike that delicate balance between encouraging the nurses to consider how things could be done differently in the future and encouraging them to move on. However, in encouraging reflection some of the questions and areas explored may feel confrontational. It is important to remember that the clinical supervisor does not set the agenda; rather the specific issue is being discussed because the supervisees have introduced it.

Introducing group supervision

Once the decision to offer group supervision has been made, a number of questions still need to be considered. These questions are now considered in detail.

Will the group be closed or open?

A closed group is one where the membership is decided when clinical supervision begins and is not open to any new members throughout the process. Membership generally carries the expectation of commitment to attend all sessions. An open group allows for dynamic and changing membership. Members attend as often as they can and new members can join the group as required.

Reflective exercise

- Consider the advantages and disadvantages of both open- and closed-group supervision.
- Which approach do you feel would best suit your organisation?

In reflecting you have identified some advantages and disadvantages to group and individual supervision. Closed-group supervision is likely to more readily facilitate the development of a trusting relationship and therefore allow the group to work towards achieving team goals. An open group may find it difficult to enter into a working phase because group members are essentially re-establishing themselves in each session.

On the other hand, a closed group requires a commitment for regular attendance that can be very difficult to achieve. The changing membership of an open group probably more accurately reflects the realities of nursing teams. The fact that nursing relies so strongly on shift work means that the nursing team is ever-changing. The difficulties that occur with open-group supervision are therefore likely to mirror those faced by the broader team, and this approach may offer a starting point to deal with some of the issues presented by a dynamic and changing team.

An open group offers the opportunity for nurses to 'warm' to clinical supervision. As discussed earlier, clinical supervision is frequently misunderstood by nurses, and may lead them to avoid this initiative when it is first introduced. Feedback from participants may encourage them to join in at a later stage. Not only does closed-group supervision remove this option, it might contribute to preconceived ideas that clinical supervision is an elitist activity. Table 4.1 presents an overview of the advantages and disadvantages of both open and closed groups.

Table 4.1 Advantages and disadvantages of open and closed clinical supervision.

Open		Closed	
Advantages	**Disadvantages**	**Advantages**	**Disadvantages**
More accurately reflects reality of nursing teams	Can challenge development of trust	Facilitates trust more quickly with the supervisor and other group members	Particularly for nursing ward environments it is very difficult to gain commitment for regular attendance
Opportunity to mirror or parallel challenges of the broader team	Team goals can be difficult to identify and maintain	There can be a real focus on team goals	Does not reflect the dynamics of nursing teams
Nurses can try out clinical supervision once or twice without having to commit	Continual need for the group to re-establish with new or changing members	Consistency of membership generally allows members to use the time efficiently as there is less disruption as a result of admitting new members	Clinical supervision may appear as an elitist activity
Other nurses may be encouraged to join following positive feedback from others	It can take a long time for the group to move through the stages of group formation	Members move more quickly through stages of group formation	There can be envy if some members of a team are denied access

Frequency of sessions

The frequency of clinical supervision sessions will vary according to the specific needs of the group. However, group supervision should be held at least once a month. In the case of bed-based services the frequency should be increased as shift work means that some members will not be able to attend all sessions as scheduled. If sessions are held monthly and a nurse misses one, it means 2 months between sessions, which can cause loss of continuity and lessen the connection with the team. There are a number of different strategies to implement to ensure that staff members have regular access to clinical supervision. These include offering group clinical supervision sessions weekly, or offering supervision less frequently but ensuring as many staff as possible are rostered for the shift(s) where clinical supervision is held, and offering incentives (such as time in lieu) to encourage those nurses not normally at work to attend. This of course creates resource issues that would need to be managed in the overall implementation plan. However, offering supervision weekly may prove more cost-effective in the long run. Although there will be the additional costs of the supervisor for the supervision sessions, this may be cheaper than rostering extra staff for a full shift.

Duration of sessions

Group clinical supervision is generally between 60 and 90 minutes long. While it can be tempting to opt for shorter sessions to place less burden on the workplace, sufficient time is need to enable all members to contribute and become involved. In the early stages of group clinical supervision, it generally takes time for members to settle into the group, feel comfortable and begin to focus. This is unlikely to be achieved in less than an hour.

Size of group

Like all groups, the number of participants can have a substantial impact on the ability to work cohesively. Larger groups provide less opportunity for each individual to actively participate and run the risk of becoming dominated by more extravert and dominant members. Smaller groups can overcome some of these problems. In a smaller group, it is generally easier to contain the anxieties of individual members and create an environment where they feel safe enough to raise important issues. A smaller group also provides more opportunity to work constructively to address the issues that are raised.

Reflective exercise

- What size of group would you prefer? Consider the advantages and disadvantages of larger and smaller groups.
- If you were to choose a smaller group how would you determine the membership?
- Why would you choose these particular nurses and exclude others?
- What implications could this have on members of the team who are not included?
- How might you deal with these implications?

Opting for a smaller group will generally mean that some team members are not included and the group may come to be viewed by non-group members as the leadership group. This may result in resentment at being excluded or may encourage nurses not actively involved to disengage with the broader team. It may also lead to some nurses feeling they are not required to be active participants in decision-making because the leadership group can do it. Given the team focus of nursing neither of these potential outcomes is likely to be welcomed.

Larger groups may be more difficult to manage but then again may more accurately reflect reality; group clinical supervision may encourage the team to work towards addressing and resolving some of the issues that face them as a large team. By practising these skills within the group setting, it is hoped that the knowledge gained can be transferred to the work setting.

The larger the group, the greater the dynamics and activities. It can become difficult for a clinical supervisor to follow what is happening if the ratio of supervisees to clinical supervisor is too high. Ideally, the ratio of supervisor to supervisees should not be more than one supervisor to eight supervisees. In groups of more than eight a second facilitator may be needed. The decision to include a second facilitator will be influenced by the experience and confidence of the clinical supervisor and whether the group is open or closed. In a group with a more stable membership numbers greater than eight may be manageable.

Membership of the group

In addition to size, it is also important to consider who the team members are. Group supervision is often introduced for a team who work together, such as the staff of a specific ward, unit or community team. However, this need not be the case. The group may comprise nurses who hold the same role but in different parts of the organisation, for example nurse unit managers, clinical nurse consultants or graduate nurses. In this context, group clinical supervision might be used to assist members to clarify and develop their roles, identify the additional skills and knowledge they require and work towards obtaining the necessary resources to acquire these skills.

It is also very important to consider any power imbalances or 'dual' relationships in the group. The issue of dual relationships is considered in some detail in Chapter 6. However, it is also an important consideration when determining the membership of the group. It is important to consider whether there are any obvious authority issues. For example, does the nurse unit manager (NUM) or associate nurse unit manager or other staff in positions of authority attend the group clinical supervision sessions and if so what impact does this have on the group dynamics? Do staff feel comfortable raising significant issues in front of their NUM?

Group supervision can involve the whole team, including the line manager. There is no reason why the line manager should be excluded if his or her presence relates to the aim, purpose and expected outcomes of group supervision. Again it is important that these aims are clearly understood and articulated by all group members and that membership is determined and communicated from the outset. However, a line manager's presence in group supervision can be problematic for all parties concerned. For the line manager it can often be difficult to just be a participant in the group and take off his or her line management 'hat'.

For example, in group supervision the team are talking about how workload has increased and everyone is under much more pressure. One team member suggests this is because there is management pressure for shorter length of stays and increased occupancy. He states that length of stay is half what it was the year prior and the unit has admitted nearly twice the number of clients. The group nods in agreement and it appears that the team supports this member's perception. The unit manager knows that the occupancy rate is only five greater and that the average length of stay is actually 1 day longer than the previous year. There is now a dilemma between being a line manager and a peer or equal participant. To challenge this member's perception and provide accurate information to the group is important as the group can then start exploring the reasons why they have a perception they are feeling overworked and overloaded. However, the other members may react to having the perception of a peer corrected. The member who raised this issue may feel chastised or targeted by the manager and embarrassed that his boss has just corrected him in public. Other members of the group may never feel truly free to reveal their own views with the manager in the room. Some staff may even use the supervision session to raise their own profile with the manager by talking about something they did particularly well with the hope that this will be viewed positively by the manager.

The choice to have management in the group supervision sessions needs to be considered very seriously by weighing up the advantages and disadvantages.

Reflective exercise

- List the advantages of including the line manager as a member of a group for clinical supervision.
- List the disadvantages.

After carefully considering both lists do you think managers should be included or not?

Experience of the group

As for all forms of clinical supervision, knowledge of the supervisees' prior experience and expectations provides an important starting point for the process. To promote effective functioning of the group the supervisor needs to know whether the group (or its individual members) have previously received clinical supervision and if so how was that experience perceived. A more detailed overview of the information particularly useful to supervisors before commencing supervision is presented in Chapter 7. These issues are equally important for group supervision as for individuals.

The venue

Personal comfort will impact on the success of group supervision and therefore the venue becomes an important consideration. It is important that the venue has enough comfortable seating for all members and fosters communication and interaction not only between the members and the supervisor, but also between the members themselves; this usually means chairs are placed in a circle around the room. The venue must be quiet and private as interruptions will hinder open communication. A 'Do not disturb' or 'Meeting in progress' sign should be placed on the door and members should be reminded at the beginning of all meetings to turn off their mobile phones. It is particularly important to be at some distance from the workplace so that members are not able to hear what is happening on the ward or team during the supervision session. Hearing what is happening outside of the session can hinder group members' concentration and may make them feel guilty that they are not involved in direct care and are leaving all of the hard work to others.

Uses of group supervision

Group supervision can be used in a range of ways; this will be influenced by the size of the group, how well the supervisees know each other, what the nature of their relationship is and what roles supervisees have within the team or organisation. Group supervision can take on many forms, for example:

- It can focus on team functioning, how people are working together, working through and exploring the barriers and strengths of the team.
- It can be used to discuss how the group are relating and working with a client. The client may present specific challenges because:
  - his or her condition is particularly complex and presents specific challenges to staff
  - he or she has a specific medical condition or health care need that the team are not particularly familiar with
  - his or her behaviour is perceived by the team as difficult or challenging.

The approach to group supervision commonly adopted in mental health is multidisciplinary, as the work often occurs within a multidisciplinary team. This approach could, however, be used across a range of nursing specialties where a range of disciplines work closely together.

- It provides the ideal setting for role-plays and other experiential approaches to dealing with a particular situation. Group members can act out a particular scenario, with other members observing, providing feedback and offering alternative strategies. For example, some supervisees may have raised difficulties in relating to one of their patients' family members, who is very demanding and distressed. This could be an opportunity to explore alternative approaches, discover if others are having a different experience and/or gain support to deal more effectively with the situation.

- When group members work in different areas opportunity is provided for them to discuss their local issues and receive support and feedback from others who may have had similar experiences. This encourages networking and the exchange of information between peers.
- The group may be for part of a team, for example the nursing staff. The aim of group supervision may be to strengthen their collective role within the health care team, or they may have needs that are quite specific in nature that are best met through their own clinical supervision. In the mental health field, for example, the strong multidisciplinary focus can have significant implications for the professional identity of nursing, i.e. what is the specific contribution of mental health nursing to the care and treatment of people experiencing a mental illness? Such a question could be an important focus for group clinical supervision.

Group processes in clinical supervision

The forming–storming–norming–performing model of group development was first proposed by Bruce Tuckman (1965). Tuckman maintained that these four phases are all necessary and inevitable in order for the team to grow, face up to challenges, tackle problems, find solutions, plan work and deliver results. This model has become the basis for subsequent models of group development and team dynamics, and a management theory frequently used to describe the behaviour of existing teams. The Tuckman model (Tuckman, 1979; Tuckman & Jensen, 1977) can equally be applied to group clinical supervision.

This model has been represented in many ways visually; although it was originally represented in a liner format a number of other theorists have proposed cyclical models (Bales, 1953). For the authors, the liner model does not capture the fluidity of group development and group dynamics as groups rarely progress through the stages of formation in a structured way, particularly open groups. Smith (2005) has restructured Tuckman's initial model to reflect the same phases but allow for issues to recur at different points in a group's life. Figure 4.1 is an adaptation to the Smith model to include the fifth stage of the model, that of adjourning or mourning.

Forming
During this stage the group members establish boundaries, identify why they are together, and begin exploring what they hope to achieve

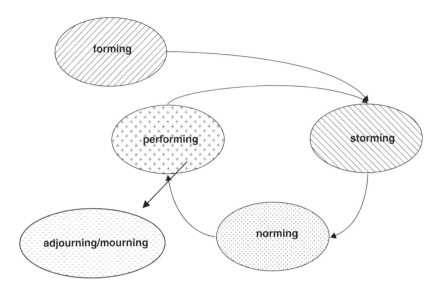

Figure 4.1   Tuckman's model of group processes.

from clinical supervision. In the early formation of groups some dependent relationships can develop. This usually occurs when group participants depend on the facilitator, or stronger members or leaders
of the group, to develop the agenda, to lead group discussion and to
manage or control the group. The group establishes the boundaries for
exploring their practice, for example whether the group will be closed
or open, the membership of the group and how regularly they will
meet. They often look to the clinical supervisor to assist in establishing
these boundaries.

Clinical supervisors take a more active role at this time, guiding and
actively facilitating while relationships develop and people feel more
able to speak without invitation. The clinical supervisor may ask questions that would enable the group to define themselves and the boundaries of the group.

Storming
As the name suggests, during this stage the group members commonly
experience conflict. It is not unusual for members to interact on an
emotional level as they tend to operate as individuals rather than as
members of the group. Some members may be resistive to functioning
as a group and focusing on the task(s) at hand. This is particularly
likely if members come unwillingly to clinical supervision. They may
be influenced by the many myths about the process (as discussed in
Chapter 1). Clashes between individual members may become a focal
point at this stage. Some members may assert themselves and test out
what can and cannot be discussed.

The role of the clinical supervisor in this stage is to manage his or her own anxiety in the face of such turmoil. The supervisor may feel overwhelmed by what is being disclosed but it is important that the group members have the opportunity to develop and express their thoughts. Containing a group does not mean that there is not any volatility; indeed it can mean more volatility. The fact that the group has confidence in the supervisor's capacity to manage group dynamics may mean that members feel more able to raise sensitive issues, resulting in a great deal of activity. The group can be volatile during this stage and the clinical supervisor may become the solid reliable ground for the members to hold onto. It is, however, a time when the supervisor may feel incompetent and powerless because of the turmoil. There may be open challenges to the role of supervisor, people may at times start scapegoating one or more members. It is an important role of the supervisor to ensure that the group is as safe as possible by not tolerating scapegoating. Putting a stop to negative behaviour can be difficult and is made easier if agreements about relating respectfully are established at the beginning of the group. It is important to be confident that the storm will pass!

In closed groups there is a more distinctive beginning and end to this stage. In an open group it may feel as though the storming phase keeps reappearing; this occurs because of the regular introduction of new staff.

Norming

This is the stage where individuals begin to function as part of the group. Roles are established and opinions voiced. The purpose of the group is identified. There is a greater sense of comfort amongst members and they begin to use the time more effectively.

The role of the clinical supervisor during this stage is more one of support by clarifying what the group has agreed on. The group should be feeling more comfortable together and therefore better able to cope with more probing questions from the supervisor regarding the focus of the work they have agreed to do.

Performing

During this stage the group members are energetic and working towards the completion of the task. Members now have established roles, they work through the issues creatively and flexibly. At the commencement of each session they quickly get down to work, they know how to use the time and they work well together. They interact well as a group, not looking for the clinical supervisor to drive things. When the group is functioning well the members may not be thinking of the group ending. It is opportune during this phase to consider the finishing point (if there is one).

As the group is functioning effectively the role of the clinical supervisor is much less active. He or she may provide input when it is needed to continue the flow or add something they have noticed as information that may benefit the group. While the group is relating well and engaged in meaningful discussions, the clinical supervisor will not want to interrupt the flow.

Adjourning or mourning

Bruce Tuckman subsequently refined his theory and added a fifth stage to the forming–storming–norming–performing model – he called it adjourning. This has also been referred to as deforming and mourning. Adjourning is arguably more of an adjunct to the original four-stage model rather than an extension. This stage views the group from a perspective beyond the purpose of the first four stages. The adjourning phase is certainly very relevant to the people in the group and their well-being, but it is not part of the main task of managing and developing a team, which is clearly central to the original four stages.

This stage occurs as the group comes towards its conclusion. Group members explore the impending end and review or finish their work. It is important that consideration is given to the 'What now?' question. For example, if a task has been achieved, how will it be sustained or improved upon? What processes need to be put in place to ensure this happens? What resources are required and how will they be secured? It is possible that the group members may experience some grief as the process comes to a close. It is important that this be acknowledged and dealt with.

The role of the supervisor during this stage is to assist the group to deal with the ending. This means not allowing group members to collude in silence, pretending it is not happening. The supervisor will raise the pending end of the group a few weeks beforehand, ensuring there is time for the members to consider how they feel about it. The clinical supervisor may, depending on the type of group, facilitate an activity or leave a structured part of the group to work with the issues related to ending. Some of these might involve exploring the journey of the group or talking about how the group has been for the members. Did they feel that they had achieved what they were hoping to? Are there any goodbyes to each other as well as the group as a whole?

Tuckman's model may be seen to present the best case scenario. Of course not all groups function as effectively and cohesively as the five-stage model depicts. Groups may not flow through each stage, i.e. some may storm frequently, others may not have a defined ending.

Five basic assumptions

Lawrence *et al.* (1996) identified five basic assumptions, adding to the work of Bion (1961), who developed the first four. These are not necessarily good or bad, they are behaviours to be aware of that can help us understand how the group is functioning. These can commonly occur and are:

(1) fight/flight
(2) pairing
(3) oneness
(4) dependency
(5) me.

Fight/flight

This occurs when members consider the group to be more important than individuals. Members are ready to either attack or withdraw. For example, when a contentious issue is being discussed the group joins to attack the individual who raises the point or prepares to walk out or silently withdraws, therefore avoiding the discussion.

A fight or flight assumption may threaten the safety of the group. No-one will feel safe if it is possible to seriously attack a member. It can feel as though the group is lacking containment when fight/flight is at play. The role of the supervisor in this situation is to provide containment, redirecting to healthier relating where possible, sometimes naming what is difficult to name in a group that is silent and not communicating.

Pairing

This occurs when group members believe in the possibility of two members providing security. For example, the group listens to the discussion of a couple of members. The group believes these individuals carry the ideas, hope and energy for the group. The other members defer to this pair and await the answer or decision.

Pairing may present a barrier to group clinical supervision if it negates the function of the team. Where two individuals are seen as the drivers and decision-makers, other members may not become active participants. There may be other times when this type of group function poses no risk; it is simply something to be noticed. The destructive elements come in to play when the group is focused on this way of relating. The role of the clinical supervisor is to closely observe if the group is focused on the pair and if so they may need to facilitate other members reconnecting, for example by asking the opinion of other members about what is being discussed and posing specific questions to other members. Alternatively there may not be a need to intervene, the discussion may be useful and provide the opportunity for the group to start contributing and commenting on what is being said without a specific intervention being necessary.

Oneness

This describes the situation when all (or at least the perception that all) group members are united around the same issue. For example, they support each other and are prepared to defend the cause. This may be considered advantageous in many circumstances. Unions are built on oneness, people united for a cause, banding together to achieve something or to protect something that is under threat. However, oneness can be unhelpful when the group will not allow any different opinions to be voiced or explored. This will create considerable difficulties for any members of the group who have a different opinion. They may be censured by the group or may be reluctant to express differences. Given the dynamic nature of contemporary health care, the ability to hear and consider different approaches and viewpoints is imperative.

The role of the supervisor is to identify if this is occurring and if so to consider whether it is constructive or destructive. A destructive situation might be when individuals are unable to hold an opposing view that is respected by the majority. Sometimes it is necessary for the supervisor to give voice to what cannot be spoken about, that is to ask questions that will assist the group to analyse and question rather than blindly accept and agree. This needs to be done in a way that is not perceived as an attack on the group.

Example

A unit team are talking about how much they all agree with the new rostering system that allows people to elect permanent days to work. Most staff are very excited; however, there are a couple of staff not saying very much. As the clinical supervisor you are hypothesising that they do not agree with the majority of the team but do not feel comfortable voicing an opposing view. You acknowledge the position people are happy about by saying that 'It seems that people are very excited about the new system and there seem to be many advantages for people'. Then you might add, 'Having said that are there any difficulties with it? For example, some people may get less money if they never work a weekend.' In this example you are making it easier and safer to bring the less dominant position into the group for discussion.

Dependency

In this situation the group seeks and depends on a leader as a form of security and protection. In a clinical supervision group this person may be the clinical supervisor or any other member of the group who is perceived as offering some form of leadership at the time. The group passively accepts the voice of this person and follows them, rather than questioning or discussing what she or he says. In a similar manner to pairing, dependency can pose a barrier to group formation and if allowed to continue it can negate the purpose of the group and prevent it focusing on the task at hand. The role of the clinical supervisor is to assist other group members to question and express their thoughts rather than follow passively.

Me

This describes the situation when an individual member perceives the broader group in a negative light. In feeling threatened by the group, individuals become self-protective against the perceived threat. They are therefore not engaged and not contributing either to the group formation or to the task at hand.

The role of the clinical supervisor is firstly to be aware that this is occurring. This may require no action as the situation may change without any direct intervention from the clinical supervisor. Unless the clinical supervisor is aware of what the threat is, it is not possible to intervene. It is important that group members are confident that the supervisor can contain the group; this is particularly important for those feeling under threat.

Important issues for group supervision

Dealing with group dynamics

As outlined above, the nature of group dynamics means it is much more complex to facilitate group than individual supervision, especially when it is provided for a team.

Ethical issues

There are certain ethical issues that are inherent in all forms of supervision (as will be discussed in Chapter 6). However, some ethical issues pose particular or unique concerns within the group context.

- Confidentialiy: Maintaining confidentiality is an important consideration in group supervision (discussed more fully in Chapter 6). Breeches of confidentiality and disclosures of personal information to those outside the group can occur and the effects of this can be devastating. If members do not feel confident that what they say will remain within the group they may be reluctant to fully express their views. This is particularly challenging in open groups where new members have not established the trust of the broader group.
- Multiple roles: If you are a clinical supervisor internal to the organisation it is likely that you carry more than one role, such as the union representative. This may not obviously be a problem initially unless, for example, your supervisee is involved in an issue where he or she has been accused of bullying and the alleged victim needs you as the union representative. You are then faced with the problem of being in the position of needing to provide support for two people in two conflicting roles.
- Managing the containment so that people are not publicly scapegoated. This refers to situations where group members deliberately use group supervision as the venue to raise an issue with a

colleague, usually in a destructive, humiliating way. This has the potential to compromise the level of trust within the group and the capacity for its members to respectfully relate to each other. The role of the supervisor is to continually assert the importance of trust and respectful communication between members.

To overcome these barriers it is important to have established group rules written down (if possible) and agreed to by participants, especially in open groups that are incorporating new members.

Individual clinical supervision

As the title suggests, individual supervision refers to a one-to-one relationship between two people, the supervisee and the supervisor. The supervisee becomes the primary focus of the supervisory relationship.

As stated previously, individual supervision and group supervision have different functions, purposes and expected outcomes. The consideration of these factors (rather than economics) should determine which type of supervision is chosen.

Individuals, particularly those who are more introverted, often prefer to engage in one-to-one interactions in preference to groups. Not only might they feel more comfortable in communicating in this environment, but also they are not readily able to avoid the processes by hiding behind more vocal members. In addition, confidentiality is more easily achieved than with group clinical supervision.

Individual sessions are also more conducive to the development of a relationship based on openness, understanding and trust. There is also more time available for the supervisee to raise, discuss and work through particular issues of concern. The supervisee is more likely to take responsibility for his or her role in the process and because the supervisee is the focus of the session, he or she needs to come to supervision with problems to solve, issues to work through or ideas to discuss. This cannot be left to others as might be the case with group supervision.

Indications for individual supervision

Individual clinical supervision is particularly appropriate where:

- individuals want to spend time reflecting and exploring their own clinical practice
- individuals are experiencing conflict issues with all or most of the broader work team, for example they may come to supervision with a view to increasing their understanding of why this conflict is occurring and to develop solutions and coping strategies

- individuals would like to explore examples of good practice to understand why things are working well
- individual nurses are experiencing difficulty working with individual clients or clients with a particular diagnosis, such as borderline personality disorder or people who deliberately self-harm. They seek supervision to explore the reasons why they find this challenging and how they might overcome the associated problems in order to work more effectively with these individuals or groups.

Example

Abbey works in a young people's inpatient unit; she really enjoys her work as a mental health nurse and feels energised working with young people. Abbey is an associate nurse unit manager and a very popular member of staff who is generally seen as a role model to the junior nurses.

However, Abbey really struggles with a particular client group: young boys aged 12–15 years with an externalising disorder, namely oppositional defiant, ADHD and conduct disorder. She finds their opposition, constant challenging of her authority and persistent rule-breaking as incredibly frustrating and often perceives they are targeting her or behaving like this on purpose. Abbey thinks she has her feelings under control; she believes that she treats these clients professionally and effectively.

One particular strategy used in an inpatient unit with this client group is time out for bad or negative behaviours and positive reinforcement or rewards for good or positive behaviour. The time required in time out depends on the behaviour. Telling a staff member to 'get lost' might be 5 minutes in time out whereas throwing the work they were completing across the room and storming out of group might be 20 minutes.

One evening there were four young boys diagnosed with a conduct disorder on the ward. They had all joined together and Abbey was watching, suspicious of what they might be up to. She noticed from the nurses' station that things were really quiet. She was concerned that they might be up to no good and immediately went looking for them. She was surprised to see that they were all sitting around playing Monopoly. Abbey was impressed with how well they all seemed to be playing together. The boys groaned when they saw Abbey and asked how long they had time out for; it was immediately obvious to Abbey that these boys associated her with consequences and time out. Abbey was devastated and asked the other nurses on the shift what they thought. They all laughed and said it was obvious she hated working with those kids, everyone knew it.

Abbey decided to take this incident to clinical supervision to discuss it with her supervisor. Together they explored the incident but they also spent time reflecting on Abbey's reactions and feelings towards this type of client. After

Continued

much exploration it became apparent to Abbey that the reason she struggled with these clients was personal, they reminded her of her two younger brothers and took her back to a difficult time in her youth where she as the older sibling was left in charge to babysit two boys who constantly challenged and defied her. Once this was recognised Abbey and the supervisor explored what could be done to assist Abbey to work with this type of client in the future. They did not delve into the personal aspects of Abbey's life and the unpleasant childhood memories, rather they concentrated on identifying what physical and emotional reaction these boys triggered and how Abbey could recognise and then modify her responses. Together they also explored externalising disorders – the epidemiology, the prevalence, how it manifests and how much control or lack of control these boys had over their behaviour. They also explored other treatment strategies, in particular focusing on utilising positive reinforcement strategies rather than just punishment via time out.

While Abbey may always struggle with this client group, through supervision she was able to identify why she struggled, develop an increased understanding and even empathy for these boys, and find alternative ways of working with them.

- individuals identify specific issues in the work environment where they have difficulty separating their personal experiences and opinions from their role as a nurse. Refer back to the example of Mary in Chapter 1. Mary finds it particularly challenging to care for women who chose to terminate their pregnancies, given she is experiencing so much difficulty in conceiving. Mary might seek supervision in order to avoid her personal situation from interfering with her interactions with women who have terminated a pregnancy.
- in reflecting on their career goals and aspirations, individual nurses have identified specific skills and knowledge they need to develop. Clinical supervisors are chosen because of their expertise in the area concerned.

Example 1

John, a mental health nurse, has recently begun working as part of a community team. He is providing case management for a number of people with a long-term mental illness and associated disability. Many of these clients are frequently readmitted to hospital as a direct result of not taking their medication. Through his reading and private research, John has become aware of the benefits of motivational interviewing. He finds a supervisor with expertise in the area as a means of guidance as to how to learn, maintain and use these skills in the clinical setting.

Example 2

After 2 years working as a diabetes educator, Trudy has become frustrated by patients who do not take their medication or insulin as prescribed and do not adhere to the diet regime. She has seen a number of long-term consequences and unnecessary rehospitalisation as a result of these behaviours. A colleague tells Trudy that motivational interviewing may help reduce this problem. She seeks a supervisor to assist her to increase her knowledge and skill in this area.

Clearly this is not a goal that could easily be achieved within a group structure unless it was the shared aim of the group to attain these skills.

Reflective exercise

- What are the specific goals you would like to achieve through clinical supervision?
- In achieving these goals what would you see as the respective advantages and disadvantages of:
  ○ group clinical supervision
  ○ individual clinical supervision?
- Considering the positives and negatives of both approaches, which approach to supervision is most likely to meet your identified needs?

Internal vs external supervision

It is understandable that organisations often try to provide the majority of clinical supervision internally or in some instances employ a clinician specifically to provide clinical supervision. This is generally more economical than engaging a person external to the organisation. While clinical supervision provided internally can have successful outcomes, there are a number of factors to consider in ensuring safety and confidence for all parties concerned.

- Confidentiality: The supervisee must feel confident that what transpires within sessions will not be disclosed to other employees.
- Potential for defensiveness: The supervisee may at times discuss issues or conflicts with a staff member who is a close colleague or possibly even a friend of the supervisor. It is a natural tendency for people to want to defend those they respect and like when they perceive them to be under threat. However, to do so would

compromise the integrity of the supervisory relationship, and deny the opportunity for the supervisee to explore the issues further with a view to resolving them. The supervisor needs to manage the situation or recognise his or her inability to work effectively with this particular supervisee.

- Line management relationships must be considered when determining the supervision load for the supervisor. For example, it is extremely inadvisable for the one person to provide clinical supervision for staff members from a unit at the same time as providing clinical supervision for their manager. Inevitably issues will be raised from two opposing standpoints. For example, the manager may discuss his or her difficulties in performance managing a particular staff member and may seek support from the supervisor as to the possible ways to manage this staff member. Together they might even role-play some scenarios or feedback sessions. The supervisor may have an active role in assisting the manager, therefore if the supervisor is also supervising that staff member it may be difficult for him or her to remain impartial. The supervisor's opinion of the staff member may in fact be clouded or influenced (albeit unintentionally) by what the manager has said. In addition, the supervisor may hear two sides of the same story as the staff member may choose to bring the issues with the manager to supervision also. This makes it very difficult for the supervisor to maintain his or her role as a sounding board. The supervisor could ultimately find him- or herself in the awkward situation of holding information from both points of view and not being able to adequately support either.

- Managers may pressure the supervisor to divulge information about a particular staff member they have concerns about. For example, if a nurse is under performance review for a perceived failure to meet role expectations, that nurse's manager may feel he or she has a right to know about the content of supervision sessions. When the supervisor is a colleague of the manager, failure to provide the requested information may lead to a strain in their relationship (this example is explored in greater depth under ethical issues, see Chapter 6).

- The supervisor needs to consider where his or her own clinical supervision should come from. Supervisors who provide clinical supervision to a number of staff as a central part of their role could be well advised to have their clinical supervision externally. The situation can become very messy if a supervisor also has supervision internally. It is likely to be very difficult to find someone who is sufficiently distanced from all those who are being supervised for there not to be a conflict. It is also helpful for supervisors to have access to a person who is not immersed in the same culture to bring in a fresh perspective.

Multidiscplinary vs nursing-specific supervision

Opinion remains divided about whether clinical supervision should be obtained from someone from the same discipline or whether it is acceptable to go beyond disciplinary boundaries in order to seek the expertise required. Some health professionals hold strongly to the view that supervision should be provided by a member of the same discipline. Other disciplines, such as nursing, are not so hard and fast, and may prefer the specific expertise the supervisor can bring rather than their discipline background.

This is particularly apparent in the mental health field. Mental health professionals are accustomed to working with a multidisciplinary team. Through their working relationships, they gain an appreciation of the skills and knowledge that other professions may bring. Professional boundaries in mental health settings are also less distinct than they tend to be in many other health care settings, especially so in the community, where nurses and allied health staff tend to hold the role of case manager and therefore perform many similar functions. Because of this they are less likely to find supervision from another discipline an alien concept.

However, this practice does not need to be confined to mental health. Whether or not a person chooses a supervisor from their own or a different professional background should reflect the goals they hope to achieve from the process.

Take the example of John (Example 1). In his endeavour to develop skills in motivational interviewing, he has sought a clinical supervisor with that specific expertise. The supervisor may or may not be a nurse, but that is not likely to be a significant consideration for John. Once John feels he has developed an adequate level of competence and confidence in this area, he may choose a different supervisor based on his career goals or other issues facing him at that time. Similarly, a midwife may seek supervision from an obstetrician if he or she wants to gain specific skills in antenatal or postnatal care and treatment.

In some instances a nurse may seek supervision from more than one discipline at the same time. For example, in recent years Australia has witnessed the introduction of nurse practitioner roles. As we know, nurse practitioners undertake a number of roles that are traditionally the domain of the medical profession, such as the prescription of medication and ordering of diagnostic tests. Nurse practitioners and those aspiring to these roles would find the skills and expertise of a clinical supervisor with a medical background particularly valuable.

However, the nurse practitioner is not a doctor, and the maintenance and development of nursing skills is essential. A nurse practitioner may therefore seek medical clinical supervision from a doctor and nursing clinical supervision from a nurse.

Example

Megan is a diabetes nurse practitioner. As part of her role she is required to provide holistic care and treatment for people diagnosed with diabetes. To ensure her knowledge and skills regarding the various medications are adequate and remain current, Megan seeks supervision from an endocrinologist. Megan remains very clear that she is a nurse and wishes to maintain this professional identity. She is also aware of the importance of her teaching role and feels she could increase her abilities in this area. She therefore also seeks supervision from an experienced diabetes educator.

Clinical supervisory relationships can also be established between nursing specialty areas, where a nurse looks for particular knowledge and expertise that is not commonplace in his or her own field.

Example

Brendan is a midwife. He is well aware of the prevalence of postnatal mental illness. He does not believe he has the skills required to detect the early onset of these illnesses, and does not feel confident in caring for women with a postnatal mental illness. Brendan seeks clinical supervision from a mental health nurse who has specific experience in postnatal depression and attending to the psychological needs of the patients.

Conclusion

Making the decision to implement clinical supervision in many ways represents the beginning of the process. There are a number of approaches to clinical supervision, including individual and group clinical supervision, which each have advantages and disadvantages that need to be carefully considered before making a final decision. Clinical supervision can also be provided by staff members from the organisation or by someone external. Again there are a number of fors and againsts for each choice, but frequently the choice is influenced by economic considerations. Finally, there are times when nurses may find supervision with another nurse valuable, while on other occasions the most appropriate supervisor may be from another discipline. For all of the approaches described in this chapter, emphasis should be on finding the most appropriate supervisor rather than following predetermined rules.

References

Bales, R.F. (1953) The equilibrium problem in small groups. In: Parsons, T., Bales, R.F. & Shils, E.A. (eds). *Working Papers in the Theory of Action*. Glencoe, IL: The Free Press, pp. 111–161.

Bion, W.R. (1961) *Experiences in Groups*. New York: Basic Books.

Lawrence, W.G., Bain, A. & Gould, L.J. (1996) The fifth basic assumption. *Free Associations*, 6(1, no. 37), 28–55.

Smith, M.K. (2005) Bruce W. Tuckman – forming, storming, norming and performing in groups. *The Encyclopaedia of Informal Education*. Accessed November 2007 from: www.infed.org/thinkers/tuckman.htm.

Tuckman, B.W. (1965) Developmental sequence in small groups. *Psychological Bulletin*, 63, 384–399.

Tuckman, B.W. (1979) *Evaluating Instructional Programs*. Boston: Allyn & Bacon.

Tuckman, B.W. & Jensen, M.A. (1977) Stages in small group development revisited. *Group and Organizational Studies*, 2, 419–427.

Models for clinical supervision 5

Introduction

As a formal process, clinical supervision requires a structured interaction between two (or more) individuals that is directed towards the achievement of specific outcomes. Models have been developed specifically for clinical supervision; however, some supervisors prefer to adapt other therapeutic or nursing models for use in this environment. This chapter will include an overview of the following:

- the importance of models for clinical supervision
- an overview of models commonly used in clinical supervision.

It is not possible to cover all possible models in this chapter but a brief introduction to the following is provided:

- psychoanalytic
- systems psychodynamics
- reflective practice
- Kadushin
- Proctor
- Peplau
- solution focused.

The importance of models for clinical supervision

The relevance of a model is sometimes not clear to nurses who seek clinical supervision, after all supervision is supervision isn't it? Reference to models may seem overcomplicated, and the fact that many of the models used by supervisors originate from a therapeutic framework may intensify concerns that clinical supervision is really about therapy or perhaps just 'psycho-babble'.

As people we are all different, we all have our ways of examining, interpreting and making sense of the world we live in. Our approaches to our work and our relationships are influenced by the attitudes, views and opinions we hold. We have different approaches to problem-solving and solution-seeking.

Reflective exercise

You are in an ambulance on your way to hospital following a car accident. You have a broken femur and facial lacerations. Your partner is midway from Australia to the UK on an important business trip. The following things keep running through your mind:

- The kids are due to be collected from school in 2 hours' time.
- Will I end up with one leg longer than the other?
- How bad are my facial injuries? What am I going to look like now?
- The unit I work in is already short staffed, how will they cope without me?

Now imagine you could automatically conjure up three people to help you deal with your current situation:

- Who are they?
- Why did you choose these three people?
- What would you want them to do?
- Why do you think they are the best placed to take on these roles?

Of course, different people will respond to this question differently. You may only want one person to take care of everything, but you also might want three different people. You may have chosen one person to look after your children because he or she is dependable, available and has a good relationship with them. You may have chosen someone else to contact your partner and your workplace because he or she is calm, reliable and tactful. You may have chosen another as someone to talk to because he or she is a good listener, or because you can rely on him or her to give you the truth.

There are two main points to this exercise:

(1) We often choose different people to provide different types of assistance when we are in need.
(2) We choose people to help and support us based on our own values and opinions about how we want things to be done.

The same rules apply to the selection of a clinical supervisor. In order to get the maximum benefits of clinical supervision the supervisee needs a supervisor he or she can work with effectively. For example, a person who does not like role-plays would be unlikely to choose to work with a clinical supervisor who uses a psychodrama framework. Such a mismatch is likely to cause frustration for both parties and may result in the supervisee not only disengaging, but also subsequently concluding that clinical supervision is a waste of time. However, it is important to note that a clinical supervisor will facilitate a process, not 'do everything'. It is about psychological containment and support for all elements of the supervisee work environment, the good as well as the difficult.

The first step towards selecting a supervisor involves developing a familiarity with the models and approaches available, and then reflecting on your own learning style and the way you prefer to solve problems and identify solutions. This should assist you in determining the model of supervision that best suits your needs and assist you in finding an appropriate supervisor.

In the remainder of this chapter an overview of popular models of clinical supervision is provided. We commence with the psychoanalytic model and systems psychodynamics because these approaches underpin much of the clinical supervision process irrespective of which model is used.

The psychoanalytic model

This theory has had a significant influence on the development of therapeutic approaches and our understanding of how we relate to one another as individuals. It can therefore be particularly helpful in increasing our understanding of how we, as nurses, relate to our colleagues and our patients. Whilst it will be presented as an actual model, the concepts raised in this section are applicable to all supervision sessions and can be adopted for use regardless of what model you choose.

Overview

When the term 'psychoanalysis' is used, it frequently conjures up an image of the patient lying on the couch, talking about traumatic events recalled from childhood or responding to random words through free association. The suggestion of having clinical supervision from a psychoanalytic approach might be very off-putting to many nurses; they may not be aware of what the approach has to offer.

It is not within the scope of this book to provide a highly detailed description of psychoanalytic theory, but it is important to clarify its potential function and purpose for clinical supervision. Psychoanalysis is complex, and the therapists trained in this discipline study for long periods of time and engage in their own therapy for a number of years as part of a rigorous preparation for the role. We will refer to some of the key elements of the model rather than providing a comprehensive description of it.

The model itself focuses on understanding mental processes and exploring the unconscious world. The unconscious may be accessed through the interpretation of dreams, symbols, free associations or 'Freudian slips'. Freud believed that one of the most motivating drives for people was to avoid tension, most often manifesting in anxiety. The psychoanalytic supervisor provides a consistent work space for the supervisee by meeting at the same time of the week, with the same supervisor in the same room. This assists the supervisee to start the work (Strachey & Richards, 1991). Having consistency in the supervisory relationship also assists the supervisee to associate the time and space they have for clinical supervision as being just for them and with a specific purpose.

When used for therapeutic purposes, the psychoanalytic approach can result in the patient generating a strong dependent relationship with the therapist. Through this dependency, the individual reveals his or her deep concerns and anxieties, and these are subsequently explored through a long-term relationship (Rustin, 2001). This is one area of significant difference between the therapy and clinical supervision; the creation of dependency is not encouraged within clinical supervision.

The supervisor adopting a psychoanalytic approach must have a solid understanding of projection, transference, countertransference and parallel processes. Using this model the supervisor works with the supervisee's unconscious and conscious fantasies about their work and what they are like in their workplace.

Projection

This is a defence mechanism describe by Freud, where the feelings and thoughts are not acknowledged by the individual concerned but rather are attributed to another person (Horney, 1964). For example, a person complains about a colleague who is always running others down in public, noting their shortcomings and admonishing their professional skills. He or she proceeds to articulate the many reasons why he or she does not like this individual, accuses him or her of being a bad nurse, of being indiscrete and of failing to raise conflict issues with the specific individuals concerned directly. Clearly the behaviour he or she describes as negative in the other person is exactly the behaviour he or she is demonstrating, yet there appears to be no awareness of this. Although this may be occurring out of the awareness of the supervisee, the clinical supervisor who has an understanding of projection would recognise this is occurring and be able to overt this to the supervisee so that it can then be worked through.

Transference

This refers to an unconscious process where past experiences impact and influence the present. This is a specific form of the defence mechanism projection (Sadock & Sadock, 2007). In the clinical supervision relationship, the supervisee attributes feelings, thoughts and behaviours they have for someone else to the clinical supervisor. The supervisee projects these feelings and thoughts onto their clinical supervisor.

For example, the supervisee experiences difficulties in dealing with authority figures due to authoritarian parenting. Consequently, the supervisee adopts a defiant and uncooperative attitude towards managers. The supervisee regards the supervisor as an authority figure and finds ways to resist communicating openly with the supervisor or working constructively to develop a productive relationship.

Countertransference

Gelson & Hayes (2007) define countertransference as '. . . the therapist's internal or external reactions that are shaped by the therapist's past or present emotional conflicts and vulnerabilities (p. 25)'. So in the supervisory relationship the supervisor projects feelings, thoughts and behaviours from a relationship or an individual either in the past or from outside. The supervisor attributes these feelings to the supervisee. Taking the example above, the supervisor fits into the authoritarian role and begins directing, even ordering, the supervisee to act and behave in a different way.

Example

The supervisee regards the clinical supervisor as all knowing; he or she denies his or her own competence, and believes he or she is only able to make decisions or practice in a particular way if the supervisor has specifically recommended the course of action (transference).

The clinical supervisor is very keen to be seen as a good or successful supervisor. She or he assumes the position of being all knowing, overdoes the advice and becomes directive. Any perceived incompetence becomes the fault of the supervisee, thus reinforcing the supervisee's view that he or she is incompetent (countertransference).

Parallel process

This is a complex concept that can be enacted at a number of levels. It is largely understood to be a result of transference and countertransference. A dynamic that is occurring between a patient and a nurse may start to occur between the nurse's supervisor and the nurse him- or herself, therefore creating a parallel process. Feelings, thoughts and behaviours experienced by nurses in the relationships with patients or colleagues may be unconsciously brought into the supervisory relationship (Frawley-O'Dea & Sarnat, 2001).

For example, a supervisee may be feeling powerless in his or her interactions with a patient, nothing seems to work and any suggestions put forward are not taken up because the patient continually comments that this has been tried and failed before. This situation is discussed during clinical supervision. The supervisor makes suggestions about trying various approaches to break through the brick wall. The supervisee quickly refutes these suggestions, claiming they have been tried before without success. The clinical supervisor begins to feel powerless in dealing with the supervisee, in a similar manner to the supervisee's expression of powerlessness in working with the patient.

The following example describes how the supervisor may work with the supervisee within a psychoanalytic framework:

Example

A supervisee describes the difficulties she is experiencing in trying to establish effective clinical supervision with a supervisee:

Supervisee: I just can't work with Jane – she doesn't like me, she doesn't want to meet with me and I can't help her if she doesn't meet with me.

Supervisor: When you say she doesn't like you, what do you mean by that, how do you know?

Supervisee: She won't meet with me and when she does she doesn't want to talk about what is happening for her. She wants to end the meeting quickly.

Supervisor: When you say she won't meet with you what happens that prevents it?

Supervisee: Umm, I guess I offered an appointment to her on Mondays at 1pm and she can never make it.

Supervisor: Is that the only option you offered her?

Supervisee: I guess it was . . . I may have made it hard for her to meet with me.

Supervisor: Why do you think you may have made it hard for the supervisee to meet with you?

Supervisee: It is uncomfortable for me to work with her, so I guess I was avoiding it.

Supervisor: *Silent pause*

Supervisee: I find it hard to relate to her, I guess in some ways I don't want to.

In this interaction the supervisor is working with the supervisee to understand what is occurring in the relationship she has with her own supervisee or rather the lack of relationship. The supervisor enquires about the situation and the relationship, allowing space for the supervisee to reflect on her responses. The supervisor develops thoughts about what may be happening. In this example, the supervisee may be demonstrating projection. The supervisee does not particularly like working with this particular supervisee (Jane), but her work values suggest she should be able to work effectively with everyone. As a way of managing this she projects that Jane does not like working with her and therefore does not keep appointments. This allows her to avoid working with Jane and therefore manage her own feelings. This has occurred outside of her awareness, an unconscious process that can start to be explored through asking questions and allowing space for the supervisee to hear her own thoughts and then reflect on these responses.

Psychoanalytic concepts relevant to all clinical supervision

Shame

Shame is not always expressed in a way that is easily recognised as such. It can take on many forms, including anger, anxiety, humiliation, depression and withdrawal. People frequently experience shame in their workplace. They may feel shamed by colleagues, superiors and/or patients.

Shame can also occur within the supervisory relationship. It takes time to establish a relationship in which supervisees will risk sharing that they are feeling shamed. As a clinical supervisor it is important to be alert to the possibility that shame can occur and be prepared to inquire about the changes you have noticed and what has led to them. For example, if a supervisee appears to be irritable and becomes withdrawn during supervision, as a supervisor you should ask why and continue to (gently) probe as it is unlikely that the supervisee will respond to this question enthusiastically.

In a group setting it is much easier to shame someone. The experience is magnified in a group because a number of people have witnessed what has occurred. Under these circumstances the individual is likely to want to withdraw from the situation rather than engage in further discussion and this may lead to further shaming experiences. Shame is more difficult to work with in the group setting but it is important not to ignore it. Shame is also likely to affect other members of the group. Some may feel their colleague was attacked or not supported and may come to his or her defence. Others may want to further the person's discomfort. Others may disengage with the group because of fear that they too may be shamed.

Blind spots

The term 'blind spots' refers to things that we cannot see ourselves because they are out of our awareness. We have blind spots for a range of reasons. People may be too close to an event to see the situation clearly; they may be denying something to themselves as a means of avoiding the pain it conjures. Clinical supervisors should use their own clinical supervision as a means to identify and deal with their own blind spots. The supervisor then works with supervisees to assist them to become more aware of the areas they cannot see and therefore develop the capacity to recognise and deal with blind spots. The impact varies depending on the blind spot.

Example

You may be working with a person who has just been diagnosed with cancer and is considering the range of treatment options. In your private life your favourite aunt is also battling with cancer and has decided not to have any treatment. You find yourself assertively encouraging your patient to have aggressive treatment, without realising you are being influenced by the distress you feel because of your aunt's anti-treatment stance.

Having a blind spot is like trying to drive to a destination that is unfamiliar, without directions or resources such as a map; you think you know what you are doing and where you are going. The risks are numerous; you could run out of petrol, end up in a deserted area or be very late for an appointment. To minimise the impact in this situation you would need to recognise that you did not know where you were driving before you left rather than when you were already lost!

Interpretation/use of silence

Silence provides the opportunity for the supervisee to generate his or her own thoughts, rather than having the supervisor assume what she or he is thinking and filling in the gaps. Learning to come to terms with silence is not easy. Frequently anxiety leads the supervisor to ask questions or give suggestions rather than waiting and allowing thinking time. Clinical supervisors need to develop the capacity to manage their own anxiety, and be able to tolerate some silence in order for supervisees to develop their own thoughts and opinions about what is occurring.

Feelings

It is very important to pay attention to feelings within the clinical supervision relationship as this can allow the clinical supervisor to become aware of transference, countertransference and parallel processes. Clinical supervisors need to be aware of their own feelings. Supervisors use themselves as a tool in the supervisory relationship, and part of doing this effectively is knowing whether you are simply responding to what the supervisee is saying or whether you are responding to what they are saying as it reminds you of your own past experiences or relationships. In colloquial terms this is often referred to as 'pushing your buttons'. When strong responses are experienced in supervision, it is important to take the time to reflect on and consider why that would be happening. Is it an indicator of countertransference? For example, you may become aware that you have very strong feelings about how a patient your supervisee is discussing should be cared for.

Example

Geraldine, one of your supervisors, describes her feelings about assisting one of her patients, who is in the last stages of a terminal illness, to say goodbye to his family. Geraldine tells you the patient and family do not want a funeral. You feel a strong urge to encourage Geraldine to convince the family how important it is to have a funeral. These strong feelings are based on your personal experience. Your father did not want a funeral and you still (5 years later) experience negative feelings because you were denied the opportunity to grieve.

Systems psychodynamics

Systems psychodynamics is a discipline that has been influenced by open systems theory, group relations theory and psychoanalysis (Smit & Cilliers, 2006). The elements of psychoanalysis discussed previously are also important in working systems psychodynamically. This model is particularly useful when working with groups because the context and systemic thinking are central to this work. Some of the concepts discussed are:

- the primary task
- authority for the task
- container/contained
- working with the unconscious processes
- the five basic assumptions (discussed in more detail in Chapter 4)

Lawrence *et al.* (1996) identified five basic assumptions that can commonly occur as part of group behaviour:

- Fight/flight: This occurs when members consider the group to be more important than individuals. Members are ready to either attack or withdraw.

- Pairing: This occurs when the group believes in the possibility of two members providing security.
- Oneness: This describes the situation when all (or at least the perception is that all) group members are united around the same issue.
- Dependency: In this situation the group seeks and depends on a leader as a form of security and protection.
- Me: This describes the situation when an individual member perceives the broader group in a negative light.

The primary task

The primary task(s) refers to that which is central to the work or role of the supervisee. It is easy for people to become involved in work that is not part of their role. Reflect on your own experiences for a moment. How often do you find yourself doing things that do not really constitute nursing work? Or doing things that one of your colleagues should be doing? This practice is not usual and it is not likely that your co-workers will deter you from doing this. For example, you may have a colleague (or often more than one) who does not pay the attention to detail that you think patients deserve. In order to ensure that the best care is provided you might find yourself checking up to see if certain responsibilities have been followed through, and if not, you do them yourself. Assisting supervisees to explore their role in terms of primary tasks allows them to see where they maybe operating outside their role; with this awareness they are then in the position to decide whether they want to continue as they are or change their practice (Bain & Bain, 2002).

Authority for the task

The scope of nursing work is largely defined by legislation. However, the boundaries are not always clear, particularly as expectations can change according to the policies and procedures of different organisations. Lack of clarity can create confusion and anxiety. Not knowing what you are allowed to do or expected to do can leave you unsure of whether or not you are doing the right thing. The other possibility is that you are faced with an expectation that is clear but unattainable. A simple example may be the result of an evolving job description. Your role may have grown over time and although what you are expected to do is clear it can no longer be achieved.

Example

Denise is a nurse unit manager. As part of her role she has a budget to manage. She is told that she must stay within the budget parameters. She creates a plan

Continued

that she believes will work but finds herself very anxious when the next budget report comes showing that she has not met the targets. During the previous month a number of patients were admitted with complex needs. The need for additional staff was apparent and the associate unit managers organised an increase in the staff compliment. The expectation that Denise stay within budget was clear but also unattainable due to a higher than usual acuity level in the patients admitted.

Example

Christine arrives at work to find two of her colleagues are on sick leave. One replacement has been found but Christine has been asked to cover the workload of the other nurse as well as her own. The instruction is clear, however, her capacity to carry it out effectively is doubtful and places considerable pressure on Christine as she is faced with trying to prioritise what she will do with the knowledge that she cannot do everything required.

Systems psychodynamics emphasises the importance of supervisees working within their scope of practice, with clear authority to do so. A comprehensive understanding of the lines of authority and structures within an organisation can assist in minimising confusion and its associated anxiety.

Container/contained

This concept refers to the importance of anxiety being contained within the supervisory relationship. This applies equally to the supervisor and the supervisee. For example, if the clinical supervisor is too containing then supervisees will not be able to be creative and generate their own ideas; they may be restricted and possibly become dependent on the clinical supervisor for making decisions because of a lack of confidence in their own ability to do so. If the containment is very strong, supervisees might not raise specific issues because of concerns about how the clinical supervisor will be able to manage.

You can demonstrate this by placing one hand around your other wrist. If you hold too tight (over contained) you will restrict the blood flow. If your hold is not firm enough (under contained) the hand will easily be able to break free.

Working with the unconscious processes

The term 'unconscious processes' relates to the experiences, thoughts and feelings that are out of the supervisee's awareness. When working with unconscious processes, the clinical supervisor will be looking for what is not said but is expressed in other ways, such as in the tone of speech, body language, the issues that the supervisee does not want to talk about or the supervisor's own intuitive feelings. These can be worked with in a range of ways. It is not always necessary for you as the clinical supervisor to share with supervisees what you have observed. At times it may be useful to help supervisees explore the situation so that they can gain the awareness themselves. Sometimes it can be helpful to point out something you have noticed. It may be something you want to clarify or pose as a question to gauge a response from supervisees. To make the decision about how to work with what you have noticed you need to ask yourself what you believe would be the most helpful to the supervisee.

Example

Julie (a supervisor) asks Michael (the supervisee) to draw a representation of himself in his workplace. Michael is asked to place himself in the picture along with his colleagues to show how they relate as a group. Michael's picture is presented in Figure 5.1.

In response to the drawing, the following discussion takes place:

Julie: Can you talk me through what you have drawn here?

Michael: I have symbolised my workplace as a pond. The black cloud on the side with the fishing rod extending into the pond represents a threat to the team from outside. It is a threat that feels real but I don't know what it is; it feels like it is going to get my team.

I am the little black fish. I am closest to the threat and I am alone, swimming in the opposite direction to the rest of the fish – they are my colleagues. They don't see or feel the threat and they are swimming straight for it. I'm the team leader and I don't know how to fit with them.

The frog on the throne is my line manager; she is happy where she is. She is hard to reach and she is stuck in the middle of the pond not able to move off the throne or the lily pad, which is her office.

Julie: Why the throne?

Michael: Because she has been there a long time and thinks nothing can touch her. She offers me no support and she is also unaware of external threats.

The dark flecks in the right-hand corner are the food for the fish, which is funding and referrals. At the moment there is enough but the black cloud is coming.

Julie: There are a few things I would like to explore further with you. Let's start by looking at yourself and your team. I'm curious about why it is you feel you are swimming in the opposite direction and how does that feel?

Michael: They have also been there a long time; I'm the newest member of the team. They all feel a bit like the frog . . . protected. I don't.

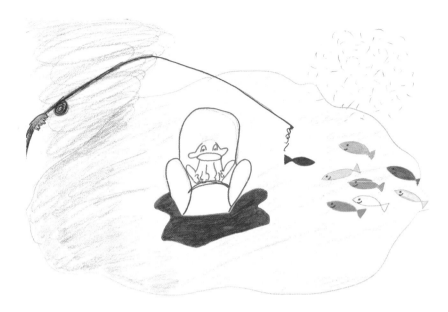

Figure 5.1   Michael's drawing.

The drawing itself can draw out unconscious processes as it has provided a medium for the supervisee to project thoughts, feelings and experiences about the workplace into a symbolic representation.

This interaction starts to capture the exploration of the drawing. Julie may be starting to think about Michael's experience in the group in terms of the five basic assumptions. Michael seems to be working from a 'me' position (feeling on his own and threatened) and the team seems to be working in 'oneness' (as described, the team all think the same way, there is uniformity). Julie may be questioning the level of containment Michael has in his role given his description of his line manager and the level of threat he perceives. This can be quite a long process that may extend over a number of sessions or be referred back to at a later stage. Similar processes can also be used working with groups, this is, however, more complex and requires considerably more time.

Reflective models

Using a reflective model for clinical supervision provides a forum for intentional reflection on practice. Nursing is undoubtedly an intense and busy profession; the demands on nurses to meet the health care needs of patients, ensure professional practice and conform to organisational policies and procedures is ever-increasing. As a result nurses often find themselves so busy doing that there is little time left for thinking. 'Reflection (rather than merely thoughtful) practice requires that nurses learn from their reflections, revise their conceptual perspectives appropriately and act differently in the future as a result' (Daly *et al.*, 2004: 279).

Despite a commonsense view to the contrary, nurses and leaders must learn how to reflect. Reflection is a purposeful, highly intellectual skill that requires effort and practice. It is neither innate nor inactive, rather reflection and reflective models are a highly interactive and active way of learning (Greenwood, 2001; Daly *et al.*, 2004).

A reflective approach to clinical supervision provides 'time out' to reflect and examine practice with the support and facilitation of a clinical supervisor. In the literature there are many models of reflection written about some time ago but that remain relevant even today (Benner, 1984; Atkins & Murphy 1993; Johns, 1997).

Essentially, reflection refers to a process that supports nurses by empowering them to more fully understand their nursing practice and how it influences and is influenced by their unique personalities. It provides the basis for the examination of nursing actions in order to identify ways in which actions are embedded, informed and transformed by different forms of knowledge. This subsequently leads to greater understanding and awareness, thereby enabling nurses to develop and even transform their practice as a result of this increased knowledge. These are essential characteristics for effective practice development (see Chapter 2).

Driscoll (2000) describes clinical supervision as a process of guided reflection, where the supervisor assists the supervisee in this process. Driscoll's 'What?' model has three main components:

- What? – a description of the event
- So what? – an analysis of the event
- Now what? – proposed actions following the event.

Each of the components identifies different stages in the process of the reflective cycle and movement through each stage in the model is supported with the use of trigger questions. The supervisor uses the trigger questions to gently guide the supervisee through a process of active reflection.

Examples of the trigger questions used at each stage include:

What trigger questions – What:

- actually happened?
- did you see/do and what was your reaction to the event?
- did other people who were involved in this event do?
- is the purpose on reflecting on this particular event?

So what trigger questions – So what:

- did I feel at the time?
- were my feelings like compared to others?
- are my feelings now after the event?

Now what trigger questions – Now what:

- are the implications for me and others in the situation?
- difference does it make if I choose do to nothing?
- can I do to modify my practice if this situation arises again?

After the 'Now what' section the supervisor and supervisee would spend time reflecting on the event and summarising what has been discussed in the session in relation to it.

If the reflections lead to a decision that something could be done differently in the future, a plan would then be formulated by the supervisee and supervisor to action the new learning. It is important to spend time discussing how the supervisee would action and what has been learnt in the session. At the following session the supervisor and supervisee would spend time reviewing and discussing how actioning the new learning actually went. A diagrammatic representation of Driscoll's What model is presented in Figure 5.2.

The model and the trigger questions are intended as a guide rather than as a prescriptive formula.

A limitation of this and other reflective models is that it is event dependent. The supervisee is required to focus on an event and bring this event to the session. This type of model is not suited to meandering discussions perhaps focused on dynamics or an exploration of the work environment/team rather than an actual event or incident.

The Kadushin model

The Kadushin model of clinical supervision was developed for use in the field of social work. A review of social work literature identifies that clinical supervision was first conceived as an essential aspect of the training of social workers by Robinson (1949). The *Encyclopaedia of Social Work* (p. 5) defines supervision as 'an educational process in which a person with a certain amount of knowledge and skill takes responsibility for training a person with less equipment'. This early definition focused on the administrative and educational functions of supervision.

It was not until the work of Kadushin (1985) that the expressive or supportive function of clinical supervision was articulated and included as an essential and necessary component to social work supervision. Kadushin argued that all three functions of clinical supervision were mandatory and complimentary. Despite these three functions being drawn as three circles of equal size, touching but not overlapping, the way the model is described is that these three functions overlap and are not necessarily of equal size and importance, and provide a holistic framework for the supervisor and supervisee. Supervisors must use their judgement and experience to determine which function of the

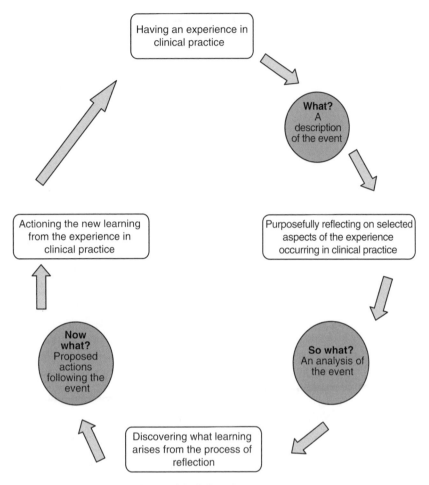

Figure 5.2 Driscoll's What model of clinical supervision.

model requires more or less emphasis in each scenario. The Kadushin model is presented in Figure 5.3.

The administrative or managerial functions are the essence of administrative supervision. The primary role of the administrative function is the effective application of the organisation's policies and procedures. It is the role of supervision when focused on this function to ensure that the supervisee is adhering to all the various legal and ethical frameworks, such as codes of conduct, policies, protocols and guidelines. This part of the model also concerns monitoring the supervisee's adherence with the organisation's administrative functions. In the administrative phase of this model regular evaluation of the supervision sessions occurs in order to ascertain whether supervision is working well.

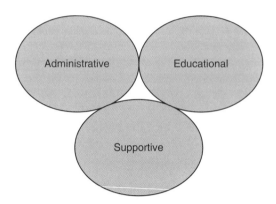

Figure 5.3   Kadushin's model of supervision.

The educational function focuses on the knowledge and skills of the supervisee. It is concerned with ensuring that the supervisee has the knowledge required to complete certain tasks. This part of the model focuses on the professional development of the supervisee. The provision of educative supervision is particularly important to skill development, the linking of theory and practice, and increasing competence, job satisfaction and hence morale for both supervisors and supervisees.

Whilst both administrative and educational supervision are concerned primarily, although not exclusively, with instrumental considerations, supportive supervision is concerned with the expressive component. It refers to maintaining the overall well-being of the supervisee. Supportive supervision provides recognition of the inherently stressful nature of the work and provides the psychological and interpersonal resources that enable the practitioner to mobilise the emotional energy needed for effective job performance and to prevent stress and burnout.

This model of supervision provides a framework or a way of looking at a scenario presented by the supervisee. Each time an issue is presented in supervision both the supervisor and the supervisee consider this issue from an administrative, an educational and a supportive perspective.

This three-pronged approach provides a well-rounded structure by ensuring that all the essential components that make up supervision are discussed. By ensuring that all three parts of the model are discussed in supervision, the session is less likely to inadvertently become line management (administrative only), an education session (educational only) or a counselling or therapy session (supportive only).

Reflective exercise

In your role as a clinical supervisor, a supervisee presents you with the following scenario from her clinical practice.

Janelle, a 17-year-old female, has been admitted to a medical ward following a major overdose with insulin. She has diagnoses of depression, borderline personality disorder and insulin-dependent diabetes. Janelle has a past history of sexual abuse, self-harm and suicidal ideation, and has had frequent hospitalisations in medical and mental health units. Janelle is described as a high-risk client. Due to the complexity of her situation there are multiple agencies involved, including the Child and Adolescent Mental Health Service (CAMHS), the Department of Human Services (DHS), the Centre Against Sexual Assault (CASA), her GP, the diabetes educator, the school nurse and the school counsellor. The supervisee is particularly concerned about the communication problems between the various agencies, resulting in lack of consistency. Janelle seems to be using this lack of communication to split her system and pit various people against one another.

As the supervisor, how would you assist the supervisee to approach this situation using the Kadushin model?

It is easy to become overwhelmed at the thought of tackling a situation such as this, particularly if you are not experienced in clinical supervision. It is important to remind yourself that you are not expected to have the answers or to solve the problem. Even if this were possible it would not be desirable. The role of the supervisor is to provide assistance, guidance and support to the supervisee as he or she develops strategies to overcome clinical challenges or problems.

In the case presented above, using the Kadushin approach you would work with the supervisee to consider the topics or discussions under each function. You may encourage the supervisee to consider the following areas.

Administrative

- Who are the services involved and what do they do? What is their role or mandate?
- Identify important policies/protocols such as who has case management? (You might want to explore legal issues here. What else might you explore?)
- How could the supervisee and you map the system? A sociogram or a social map can be drawn on the white board or butchers' paper and is a visual diagram that may help to make sense of the system. The diagram could show where relationships exist between services, and the possible conflicts and alliances between them, by

using the symbols used in a genogram. This is often a very useful tool, particularly when systems are complex. Trying to verbally describe everything that is going on can be quite confusing and challenging. Being able to visibly map or draw is often much clearer, and the supervisee then has something tangible to take away if it is helpful to do so.

A diagrammatic representation of a sociogram is presented in Figure 5.4.

The sociogram in Figure 5.4 visually identifies just how complex Janelle's system is. It identifies her family and how many services are involved. The sociogram also highlights which services are closely aligned, which services are currently experiencing conflict and which parts of the system are not connected at all. Once the supervisee has drawn this sociogram you can continue to tease out aspects of Janelle's system to explore the communication difficulties and splits.

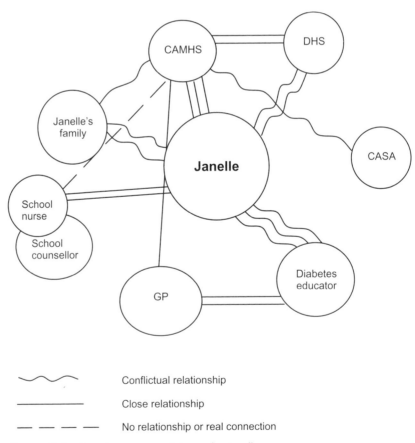

∿∿∿	Conflictual relationship
———	Close relationship
— — — —	No relationship or real connection

Figure 5.4   A sociogram or social map for Janelle.

Educational

- What are the key words or concepts, for example 'splitting' between staff and services?
- What is the supervisee's understanding of these key word concepts? As the supervisor you may have a good knowledge of these but it is important to consider the supervisee's understanding, not yours.
- What else can be gained or explored in the relationships in the system, for example power differentials between services or hidden agendas?
- What new knowledge does the supervisee need to improve her understanding of this situation?
- How can that knowledge best be attained?

Supportive

- How can or would you support this supervisee in this situation?
- How can you help the supervisee to explore her role in the splits in a supportive way?
- How is the situation affecting the supervisee in her role as a nurse? For example, the supervisee's desire to be liked may interfere with her ability to work consistently with Janelle.
- Validate the supervisee's role and insight.

Within the framework of social work clinical supervision there is no direct link with line management. The clinical supervisor is considered a middle management position, responsible for all service workers but accountable to an administrative manager. The supervisor straddles the divide between clinicians and manager without fitting into either group. The Kadushin model of clinical supervision, conceived in 1985, continues to be the predominant model of clinical supervision in social work (Mullarkey & Playle, 2001). Thus, clinical supervision in social work has tended to be uni-professional, with social workers supervising social workers (Kadushin, 1985; Mullarkey & Playle, 2001).

Proctor

The model of clinical supervision developed by Brigid Proctor is the most popular model of clinical supervision in the UK. When the National Health Service (NHS) considered implementing clinical supervision they were keen to recommend one model and train all supervisors and supervisees in this model. The Proctor model was chosen by the NHS and as a result it has been widely researched and implemented across several health trusts in the UK.

Reflective exercise

Brainstorm the advantages and disadvantages of implementing the same one model of clinical supervision across your organisation.

Research from the UK (White *et al.*, 1998) indicates that the advantages from implementing the Proctor model include:

- evaluation
- consistency
- benchmarking
- measuring quality
- ease of training.

The main disadvantages include:

- model not suited to some supervisors and supervisees
- difficulty ensuring people adhere to the model
- difficulty evaluating if people do adhere to the model
- not suited to some clinical settings.

The Proctor model is almost identical to the Kadushin model in that it consists of three main functions: formative, normative and restorative.

The formative function is similar to the educational function of Kadushin, that is the developmental role of supervision. It requires a partnership between the supervisor and supervisee which focuses on the learning and developmental needs of the supervisee. It is concerned with the identification and development of skills, and the integration of theory with practice.

The normative function equates to the Kadushin administrative function. It refers specifically to the ongoing monitoring, evaluating and assessing roles that supervision may involve. This provides the quality in supervision. The focus here is on values, beliefs, evaluation of care, documentation, policies and procedures, accountability and caseload management.

The third function, restorative, refers to the supportive function of clinical supervision. The responsibility of the supervisor is ensuring that the supervisee is adequately refreshed and supported. The supervisory relationship needs to be one in which the supervisee feels contained, received, valued, understood and able to feel safe and open enough to review and challenge him- or herself.

Like the Kadushin model, the Proctor model is not prescriptive. There is no clear place to start or to finish. The clinical scenario that the supervisee brings to supervision will influence where the session will start.

Example

David comes to supervision very distressed about an incident he witnessed between two of his colleagues. David is really wound up and emotional about the incident and finds it hard to explain what has happened. Using the Proctor model the supervisor would start in the restorative phase. By starting in this phase the supervisor can calm and contain David in order to provide an environment where he feels safe enough to explore the incident. If the supervisor started with David in the normative function, David may feel that the supervisor has ignored his emotional state and be reluctant to engage.

Unlike the Kadushin model, the Proctor model breaks down these three functions into additional subsections or functions. This provides more structure to the supervision session. The Proctor model is presented in Figure 5.5.

The formative function of the Proctor model is likely to focus on one of three areas, tasks, decisions or reflective practices. The task the supervisor and supervisee spend time on is dependent on the supervisee's needs. It may be that the supervisee wants to spend time learning a new task or tangible clinical procedures. This may involve discussing how to facilitate a psychoeducational group on an adult psychiatric inpatient unit or learning how to insert an indwelling or intravenous catheter.

The second area of formative development that supervision may wish to focus on is decision-making. Again each specialty of nursing will have its own particular examples of the sorts of decisions relevant to that work area. Given the increasing pressures and competing demands, these decisions are likely to be ethical dilemmas that will need time for careful exploration.

The third area of formative practice is reflective practice. It may be that the supervisee wants to bring a particular incident or aspect of

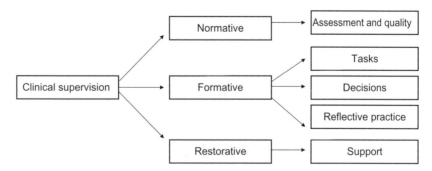

Figure 5.5 The Proctor model of supervision.

patient care to supervision to reflect on. As highlighted previously in this chapter, intentionally reflecting on a particular incident can lead to greater understanding and awareness, thereby enabling nurses to develop and even transform their practice as a result of this increased knowledge through reflective processes.

Peplau's theory of interpersonal relations

Hildergard Peplau was a mental health nurse. She developed the theory of interpersonal relations, which clearly identified the important contribution of the nurse as a therapeutic agent. Peplau's framework can be applied as a conceptual framework for the clinical supervision process. More specifically, it can provide a structure and support to the interpersonal and learning processes of the clinical supervision relationship (Peplau, 1991).

Phases of the interpersonal relations theory

The relationship is central to international relations theory, therefore the focus and awareness of the relationship development is essential during all phases.

Orientation phase

As the title suggests, this phase refers to the commencement of the supervision relationship. It is the period where the supervisor and supervisee develop a shared understanding of clinical supervision and their respective expectations. It also provides an opportunity for:

- negotiation of the boundaries of the relationship (as distinct from therapy and line management)
- confidentiality and its legal limits
- the frequency and duration of sessions
- exploration of the supervisee's goals and learning needs
- discussion and completion of the initial clinical supervision agreement.

It is important to take the time required to complete the orientation phase and not become caught up in needing to rush through the supervision in a set number of sessions. This phase sets the scene for subsequent phases and therefore is very important in establishing a successful relationship.

Identification phase

During this phase the role of the clinical supervisor is to assist the supervisee to prepare for the supervisory relationship in order that he or she can make the most of the process. It is therefore important that the supervisor:

- supports the supervisee in identifying and articulating clinical supervision learning needs and goals
- uses clarifying questions and feedback
- acknowledges the lived experience of the supervisee
- distinguishes between process and content
- acknowledges the discomfort and excitement the supervisor experiences in considering the change process that is a part of the clinical supervision experience
- supports self-knowledge on the part of the supervisee, including self-supporting strategies for managing anxiety inherent in 'working with uncertainty'.

The clinical supervisee prepares to make the most of clinical supervision by:

- recognising and articulating his or her learning needs and goals
- demonstrating a commitment to the clinical supervision process.

Exploitation phase

The name of this phase unfortunately produces some negative connotations but the intention and description of the phase is positive. Rather than referring to abuse or misuse, it refers to the operational or working phase, where the supervisee begins to use clinical supervision to work through pertinent issues and towards the achievement of the needs and goals identified in the previous stage.

The content of sessions will involve:

- exploration of the way supervisees best learn and how they can draw on their own internal resources to meet their goals
- consideration of available supports from within and external to the organisation.

The supervisee actively contributes to this stage by:

- identifying and making use of resources to assist in the attainment of goals
- regular and timely attendance at sessions, with a clear agenda for what is to be achieved during the available time
- seeking additional resources to support goal attainment, for example relevant journal articles or professional development courses to increase skill and knowledge.

The supervisor actively contributes to this stage by:

- reviewing literature and other relevant sources of information to expand own knowledge in the specific area
- utilising own clinical supervision to expand knowledge and skills in the specific area

- providing feedback on aspects of the supervisee's practice and encouraging ongoing reflection
- suggesting ways that new skills and knowledge can be incorporated into the supervisee's practice.

Resolution phase

The resolution phase applies in two ways: firstly, at the conclusion of each session and, secondly, at the conclusion of the supervisory relationship. The approach to resolution in both of these circumstances is outlined here.

The end of each session

It is important that some sense of closure occurs at the end of each session. The supervisee needs to leave with a clear understanding of what has been achieved and what needs to be done prior to the next session. Resolution therefore requires that there should be:

- A brief recap on the session and what has been achieved, for example a breakthrough in the way to manage a difficult collegiate relationship. The supervisee may have come to understand his or her contribution to the difficulty and have explored different ways to respond in the future, the need to increase knowledge base in a specific area (for example, motivational interviewing) or the identification of a particular skill or characteristic that should be enacted in the clinical situation (for example, setting limits on unacceptable behaviour).
- Identification of and agreement on 'homework' to be completed before the next session, for example meet with and talk through the difficulties in working with a colleague with a view to identifying a way forward, accessing and reading literature on motivational interviewing, or practicing limit-setting behaviour.
- A brief recap on what has been achieved since commencing clinical supervision, for example increased confidence in working with particular client groups.
- Determination of the time and date for the next session. This should never be left to 'When I have time' because nurses are busy and will never have time unless it is prearranged.
- Acknowledgement of achievements and breakthroughs.

Termination of the supervisory relationship

Ideally, clinical supervision reaches a natural ending when both parties recognise that all that can be gained from the relationship has already been gained. However, the relationship may end before this time because, for example, the supervisor is leaving the organisation. Where clinical supervision has been successful, the supervisee may develop a particularly close bond with the supervisee and the separation will therefore need to be carefully managed. The resolution phase requires the following:

- The opportunity for both parties to come to terms with the ending of the relationship and to be able to openly express their thoughts and concerns. Ideally, this should occur over a number of sessions rather than just occurring in the last one.
- The scope to review the initial goals set for clinical supervision and discuss the extent to which these have been met.
- Consideration must be given to the ongoing supervision needs of the supervisee. Will he or she continue clinical supervision? Is there someone the clinical supervisor can recommend? What other support mechanisms might be available for the supervisee?
- Identification of ways the supervisee can ensure the knowledge and skills learned during the process can be maintained and further developed.
- The opportunity to say good bye.

Strengths of the interpersonal relations theory

Peplau's phases provide a congruent structure to hold the clinical supervision process and support the growth opportunities for both the clinical supervisee and the clinical supervisor.

It includes a clear structure to assist in the organisation of clinical supervision sessions, and the basis to monitor their progress.

Because it is drawn from nursing theory this framework makes sense to nurses (particularly mental health nursing where the theory originated).

Weaknesses of the interpersonal relations theory

The framework is derived from a therapeutic interpersonal theory and may draw the clinical supervision arrangement away from its proper focus on clinical practice and into a therapeutic interpersonal domain.

The literature is limited in relation to the application of Peplau's theory to clinical supervision.

Solution-focused therapy

Solution-focused therapy is an approach based on solution-building rather than problem-solving. This is a subtle but important difference because the focal point is different. Solution-building relies on using strengths and supports to make a situation better, as opposed to problem-solving, which directs energies towards overcoming a problem. It is a future-oriented approach that emphasises current resources and future aspirations, rather than existing problems and issues from the past that may be considered to have caused or influenced them.

When people perceive problems they often tend to dwell on them, sometimes to the point of becoming obsessed, and consequently they can become overwhelmed and unable to see any way out of the situation. The solution-focused approach assumes that all people have the strength and ability to find solutions to many, if not all, of their problems and that this can best be achieved by identifying what supports are available rather than lamenting the supports they do not have.

Unlike many other approaches, solution-focused therapy assumes that the cause of the problem is not important in the discovery of solutions. Indeed, the time spent interpreting and understanding the past can be time wasted and may possibly be detrimental.

Central to solution-focused approaches is the need for the individual to be clear about his or her future goals. When these goals become clearer, it is easier and more likely that they can ultimately be achieved (de Shazer, 1998).

Similarly de Shazer (1998) argued that finding appropriate solutions requires changes in perceptions, patterns of interacting and living, and meanings that are constructed within the client's frame of reference, rather than identifying issues to be solved by therapists.

Assumptions of solution-focused therapy

- What we talk about determines what we think about. This suggests that when we talk through a problem we become more focused on it. This contradicts the essence of many other approaches that describing our problems can have a therapeutic or cathartic effect, and indeed 'holding them in' can cause them to fester or to surface in other ways such as through illness.
- Talking about the problem makes it bigger. Again this contradicts the popularly held belief that 'a problem shared is a problem halved'. On the contrary the solution-focused approach proposes that in talking about problems they assume more importance and their impact on us increases in magnitude.
- Talking about failures or deficits makes them bigger. This point assumes that when people articulate their problems, there is generally some sense of personal failure involved. For example, the person might feel some recrimination because 'I let the situation actually happen!', because 'I could not or cannot solve the problem!', because 'I let it get this big'. This therefore highlights the person's inabilities and weaknesses rather than emphasising capabilities and strengths.

- The solution-focused approach is based on the premise that people's lives are dynamic, they experience change on a constant basis. Problems are also dynamic and can be changed.
- As people we are continually influenced by our past, present and future, and the way we perceive each of these will depend on a number of other factors, such as mood or state of health. We know from our own experience that we have good and bad days. On a good day, we feel the world is a beautiful place, nothing seems too much trouble and we are generally confident that everything will be okay, workloads seem manageable and problems appear minor. On a bad day, we can feel overwhelmed with expectations and demands that seem impossible to meet, the future looks bleak and nothing can seem to shake our negative feelings. This means that our focus can change and can be changed and therefore developing solutions is within our grasp.
- The future exists in our anticipation of how it will be. If we perceive it negatively it is likely to be negative, but a more positive orientation is likely to produce a more positive outcome. Once we focus on what we want, rather than on what is wrong, we are much better placed to work towards achieving our goals.

Problems vs solutions

We construct problems by identifying and interpreting aspects of our lives as unwanted and that we wish to change. Through continuing to acknowledge our problems we effectively sustain them. Conversely, we identify and attain solutions by changing how we interpret and describe our lives (de Shazer, 1998).

The solution-focused approach in clinical supervision

In a solution-focused clinical supervision relationship the supervisor assumes the solutions already exist in the life of the supervisee; they just need to be identified. The supervisor will therefore continually encourage supervisees to focus on two main things:

- their goals
- the strengths and resources they already have that can help to make these goals a reality.

Supervisees must define and take responsibility for their own goals and keep their attention on those things that can be changed, letting go of the things that cannot. Supervisors affirm these goals and continue to remind supervisees of their successes, strengths and resources as they emerge through conversation. Furthermore, they actively discourage supervisees from dwelling on problems by bringing them back to goals and aspirations.

Example

Supervisee: I just can't seem to say no. There are a couple of people I work with who keep asking me to do extra things, things they should be doing. I know the more I keeping doing them the more they will ask me but I just can't say no.

Supervisor: Tell me how you would like the situation to be.

Supervisee: I'd like to be stronger, to be able to say 'I'm sorry I can't do that, I have my own work to do.'

Supervisor: Tell me about situations in your life when you have that strength.

Supervisee: Umm, I guess I do with my kids. They are always asking for things but when I think they don't deserve it I tell them no.

Supervisor: See, you have the ability to say no, you just need to apply that same strength in your workplace.

Supervisee: But these people I work with . . .

Supervisor (interrupts): At times your kids must have put you under quite a bit of pressure to get what they want; perhaps you could tell me more about how you were able to say no to them.

In this interaction you can see how the supervisor encourages the supervisee to identify a strength and to keep it at the forefront rather than allowing the supervisee to slip back into the problem and become overwhelmed by it. The supervisor is keeping the focus on what the supervisee has done well, saying no to the kids, rather than what has not been done well, not being able to say no to colleagues.

The supervisor using a solution-focused approach may ask the supervisee to consider the following scenario.

Suppose that one night while you were sleeping there was a miracle and this problem was solved. How would you know? What would be different? How will others know without you saying?

Because these questions require imagination rather than reality, it is often easier for the supervisee to respond without being preoccupied with 'Yes, buts' that reflect their current feelings of hopelessness and helplessness. The answers provide a concrete image of what the solution state will be like. Exploration of the answers and how they can become a reality becomes the focus of clinical supervision sessions.

What model should I use?

When you think about this chapter and the diversity of models of clinical supervision, which ones appeal to you? What models appear to suit you and your style or do you have another model of practice that you would convert for use in clinical supervision, such as a systems approach or Gestalt?

Perhaps you might like to explore one of these models in further detail, as this chapter has only been an introduction and certainly has not provided you with everything you need to practice the model exclusively and proficiently.

If you are still wanting/needing to explore additional models, Chapter 8, on clinical supervision in action, introduces a model by two of the authors of this text, the Hancox/Lynch model of clinical supervision. This model provides a framework for clinical supervision and if you are a beginning clinical supervisor you may find it useful in providing a sound structure for commencing clinical supervision in a different way from the other models in this chapter.

Do not despair if you do not find the one model that completely suits your style. Models can be adapted and used for some circumstances but not all. It is quite common for clinical supervisors to use the aspects of a model they find helpful and not use those that do not. It is more important to adapt the model to suit your approach than to adapt your approach to suit the model.

However, whatever model you choose, whatever model you gravitate towards, the relationship between the clinical supervisor and the clinical supervisee is the most important part of supervision. This supervisory relationship is paramount and needs to be nurtured, cared for and developed. You cannot avoid the concepts discussed earlier in this chapter under psychoanalytic/socioanalytic processes.

Clinical supervision is likely to become an established part of practice. The profession needs to develop a concept of the important elements of clinical supervision as they apply to nursing and then develop appropriate models for its implementation. There is no one model of supervision that will suit the needs of the great variety of clinical situations found within our profession. An attempt to impose one model that works in one area on another may have many disadvantages (Fowler, 1996; Cutcliffe *et al.*, 2001; Sloan & Watson, 2002).

Conclusion

Clinical supervision is a relationship that needs to be guided and developed according to a particular orientation or philosophical stance. In general, this means that clinical supervisors will base their approach to practice on a particular model. There are a number of models that have been developed for or adapted for use in clinical supervision. While it is not possible to cover all possible models, an overview of some of those most commonly used has been provided.

References

Atkins, S. & Murphy, K. (1993) Reflection: A review of the literature. *Journal of Advanced Nursing*, 18, 1188–1192.

Bain, A. & Bain, J. (2002) A note on primary spirit. *Socio Analysis*, 4, 98–111.

Benner, P. (1984) *From Novice to Expert: Excellence and Power in Clinical Nursing Practice*. Menlo Park, CA: Addison Wesley.

Cutcliffe, J., Butterworth, T. & Proctor, B. (2001) *Fundamental Themes in Clinical Supervision*. London: Routledge.

Daly, J., Speedy, S. & Jackson, D. (2004) *Nursing Leadership*. Marrickville, NSW, Australia: Elsevier, Churchill Livingston.

de Shazer, S. (1998) *Investigating Solutions in Brief Therapy*. New York: WW Norton.

Driscoll, J. (2000) *Practicing Clinical Supervision. A Reflective Approach*. London: Harcourt.

Fowler, J. (1996) Clinical supervision: What do you do after saying hello? *British Journal of Nursing*, 5(6), 383–385.

Frawley-O'Dea, M.G. & Sarnat, J.E. (2001) *The Supervisory Relationship, A Contemporary Psychodynamic Approach*. New York: Guilford Press.

Gelson, C.J. & Hayes, J.H. (2007) *Countertransference and the Therapist's Inner Experiences: Perils and Possibilities*. London: Routledge.

Greenwood, J. (2001). Writing nursing writing ourselves. In: Chang, E. & Daly, J. (eds). *Preparing for Professional Nursing Practice: An Introduction*. Sydney, Australia: MacLennan & Petty.

Horney K. (1964) *New Ways in Psychoanalysis*, New York: Norton Paperback.

Johns, C. (1997). Becoming an effective practitioner through guided reflection. PhD Thesis, Open University Press.

Kadushin, A. (1985). *Supervision in Social Work*. (2nd edn). New York: Columbia University Press.

Lawrence, W.G., Bain, A. & Gould, L. (1996) The fifth basic assumption. *Free Associations, Psychoanalysis, Groups, Politics, Culture*, 6(Part 1), 28–55.

Mullarkey, K. & Playle, J. (2001) Multi professional clinical supervision: Challenges for mental health nurses. *Journal of Psychiatric and Mental Health Nursing*, 8, 205–211.

Peplau, H. (1991) *Interpersonal Relations in Nursing: A Conceptual Frame of Reference for Psychodynamic Nursing*. New York: Springer.

Robinson, V. (1949) *The Dynamics of Supervision Under Functional Controls*. Philadelphia: University of Pennsylvania.

Rustin, M. (2001) *Reason and Unreason: Psychoanalysis, Science and Politics*. London/New York: Continuum International Publishing Group.

Sadock, B.J. & Sadock, V.A. (2007) *Kaplan & Sadock's Synopsis of Psychiatry*. Philadelphia: Lippincott, Williams & Wilkins.

Sloan, G. & Watson, H. (2002) Clinical supervision models for nursing structure, research and limitations. *Nursing Standard*, 17(4), 41–46.

Smit, B. & Cilliers, F. (2006) Understanding implicit texts in focus groups from a systems psychodynamics perspective. *The Qualitative Report*, 11(2), 302–316.

Strachey, J. & Richards, A. (eds) (1991) *Sigmund Freud – Introductory Lectures on Psychoanalysis*. Hammondsworth: Penguin.

White, E., Butterworth, T., Bishop, V., Carson, V., Jeacock, J. & Clements, A. (1998) Clinical supervision: insider reports of a private world. *Journal of Advanced Nursing*, 28, 185–192.

Legal and ethical issues in clinical supervision

Introduction

Nursing is an intensely personal profession. Nurses engage with patients at an extremely vulnerable time in their lives. Many ethical issues and dilemmas arise in this context and, like other professions, nurses are required to practice within a legal framework. Clinical supervision is similarly personal and encompasses a range of ethical issues. There is, however, no specific legislation that pertains to clinical supervision, but broader legal principles are relevant to this practice. The aim of this chapter is to:

- provide a brief overview of the Australian legal system
- discuss the legal implications for clinical supervision, duty of care, negligence and vicarious liability
- consider the implications of dual relationships within clinical supervision
- discuss the importance of confidentiality
- consider ethical issues and ethical dilemmas
- consider the issue of mandatory vs voluntary participation in clinical supervision.

Brief overview of the Australian legal system

Legal frameworks govern our practice as nurses. You are no doubt already aware of the numerous Acts of Parliament that influence nursing practice. Clinical supervision is not immune from the law; however, the specific relationship between clinical supervision and the law is not clear. Furthermore, in the absence of specific guidelines to govern the practice of clinical supervision, supervisors and supervisees must refer to the current legal frameworks for guidance.

In order to understand these legal frameworks we present a brief overview of the Australian legal system.

The Australian legal system has developed from the days of British colonisation, therefore we have adopted many of the legal principles from the British system. For example, the two primary approaches to making laws are:

- parliamentary law
- common law.

Parliamentary law

As the name suggests, these are the laws made in parliament. They are the written and formally recognised laws. They are Acts of Parliament; they may also be referred to as legislation or statutes.

In Australia's federated system we have Commonwealth or Federal Acts and State or Territory Acts of Parliament.

Health care is primarily governed at state and territory level. There are many examples of State Acts, known as Principal Acts, and many of these Principal Acts have subsequent amendments that directly affect nursing and health care, including:

- Drugs and Poisons Act
- Nurses Act
- Medical Treatment Act
- Health Records Act (replacing Freedom of Information)
- Child and Young Persons Act
- Mental Health Act
- Guardianship Act
- Occupational Health and Safety Act
- Equal Opportunity Act.

Some Acts of Parliament also have a second document known as Regulations. While the Act itself provides broad parameters and principles for the law, 'The Regulations generally give precise directions which must be followed in order to comply with the intent of the Act' (Staunton & Chiarella, 2003).

For example, the Drugs, Poisons and Controlled Substances Act of Victoria (1981) also includes a set of regulations.

State and Territory Acts may share many common principles with one another but they also vary and the specific requirements for each jurisdiction must be understood so that the implications for clinical supervision relationships can be appreciated.

For further information regarding relevant legislation go to:

Australian Capital Territory: www.legislation.act.gov.au
New South Wales: www.legislation.nsw.gov.au
Northern Territory: www.nt.gov.au
Queensland: www.legislation.qld.gov.au
South Australia: www.legislation.sa.gov.au
Tasmania: www.thelaw.tas.gov.au
Victoria: www.legislation.vic.gov.au
Western Australia: www.parliament.wa.gov.au

Judicial or common law

The concept of common or judicial law has developed from the under-standing that the written word will always require some form of inter-pretation. No piece of legislation can ever be written with sufficient clarity to precisely define the actions or behaviours it is intended to regulate.

There is therefore a need for interpretation of the written law when the actions or behaviours vary or divert from the written law. When judges make interpretations about the law, this is known as the doc-trine of precedent. Precedent represents a legal decision that is binding on any court that is lower on the hierarchy for that jurisdiction. For example, a decision made in the Supreme Court of New South Wales will be binding for the county and magistrates' courts of New South Wales. The county or district and magistrates' courts of other jurisdic-tions may be influenced by such a decision but they are not bound by it.

The two main forms of law in Australia are criminal law and civil law.

Criminal law refers to the regulation of specific actions and behav-iours to protect the safety and security of people. Violation of this law results in punishment, and criminal behaviour is regulated by the police force. Criminal laws define unacceptable behaviours against the person, such as murder and rape, and against property, such as theft.

Civil law refers to the resolution of disputes between people that they are unable or unwilling to resolve themselves. Civil law does not fit within the responsibility of the police force. You will quite likely have seen signs on properties stating something to the effect of 'Tres-passers will be prosecuted'. This statement is not accurate. Trespass is a civil law issue and as such civil action (commonly known as suing) would need to be taken to resolve this issue. Unless a criminal act such as theft or assault is occurring on the premises, the police and law courts will not become involved.

Civil law

The legal issues affecting nursing practice generally fit within civil law. The following civil issues are particularly relevant for nursing practice and therefore clinical supervision:

- negligence
- consent
- trespass against the person.

Negligence

Negligence refers to causing damage to another because of a failure to exercise reasonable care. For negligence to be found four elements must be observed (commonly referred to as the four Ds):

(1) Duty of care: the existence of a relationship that involves a duty of care by one person to another must be substantiated.
(2) Dereliction of duty of care: the expected or required standard of care was not provided.
(3) Damage, as demonstrated by loss or injury. This can be physical, psychological or economic (i.e. loss of income or earning potential).
(4) Direct – cause and effect: the breach caused or materially contributed to the damages suffered.

A claim of negligence will not be successful unless all four criteria can be demonstrated.

Duty of care

As nurses you are no doubt familiar with this term. We know that we have a professional obligation to provide safe, high-quality care to those who receive our services.

You may not know the origins of this concept. It may surprise you to know that it did not originate from the health care system, but rather arose from an everyday life incident.

The Donoghue vs Stevenson case is famous in legal circles. A lady (Donoghue) drank a bottle of ginger beer bought for her by a friend. After consuming most of the contents from the opaque bottle, the decomposed remains of a snail became evident. Donoghue took legal action for damages because she experienced shock and severe gastro-enteritis. One of the particularly interesting features of this case is that according to existing civil law Donoghue did not have any legal basis for successful legal action. Had she purchased the ginger beer herself she could have sued for breach of contract as the goods she purchased were not what one could reasonably expect to receive. However, she was not party to a contract. The friend who purchased the offending ginger beer could not sue because he did not experience any untoward effects.

Indeed, the original legal action undertaken by Donoghue was not successful for this very reason – the absence of a contract. The prevailing legal argument from the appeal was that manufacturers have a duty of care to ensure that goods intended for consumption must indeed be suitable and safe for consumption. Should the manufacturer fail to ensure safety, then negligence has occurred.

Determining whether or not a duty of care exists depends on two main factors: foreseeability and promiximity. Foreseeability means that people must take reasonable care to avoid acts or omissions that might reasonably be likely to cause injury to a neighbour. In this legal sense, the term 'neighbour' is not limited to the person next door or living in the same street but rather refers to persons who are sufficiently close to be directly affected by acts or omissions. In the case of Donoghue vs Stevenson, Donoghue was regarded as a 'neighbour' of the manufacturer. Clearly the acts or omissions that led to the decomposed snail being in the ginger beer could be foreseen as potentially detrimental to whoever drank the ginger beer.

In the case of nurses, patients represent the obvious neighbours as they can readily be affected by the acts or omissions of nurses. For example, if a nurse does not administer prescribed medication (omission) or administers twice the dose of the prescribed medication (act), the patient may experience a deterioration of physical condition or even death. As a 'neighbour' the patient is affected by the act or omission of the nurse and the nurse has breached his or her duty of care.

Dereliction of duty

Where legal issues arise, the courts will consider the following in determining whether or not a duty of care has been breached:

- whether the standard of care provided is what would be expected from a 'reasonable' nurse
- whether the relevant legislation has been breached
- whether there has been a breach in relevant policies and procedures.

The use of the term 'reasonable' is common within legal circles. It focuses primarily on what actions or behaviours could be reasonably expected in particular circumstances. Although it is very difficult to define exactly what is meant by reasonable, in the case of nursing it refers to what we would describe as professional standards of behaviour. Given the examples above, one might be justified in expecting the nurse to administer the medication at the dose prescribed and at the correct time. Failure to do so might indicate the breach of a duty of care but mitigating circumstances may be considered by way of explanation.

Example

Take the nurse who does not administer the prescribed medication. An explanation that he or she forgot would probably not be accepted in a court of law. Legal interpretation is likely to suggest that a 'reasonable' nurse should not forget or, stated another way, it is the expectation of patients that they will be provided with safe care, including the accurate and timely administration of medication.

Alternatively, consider the following situation. Shaun is the registered nurse in charge of the afternoon shift in a busy medical unit. Jennifer, a 16-year-old girl, is admitted with the acute onset of type 1 diabetes. The treatment orders for Jennifer include blood glucose levels and a sliding scale order for insulin, four times a day. The next time is 4pm. At 3.45pm, a new patient is admitted with an acute phase of chronic obstructive airways disease. He is an older person who is clearly very ill and requires significant attention. At 3.55pm a patient on the ward experiences a cardiac arrest. All ward staff become involved in the resuscitation efforts. At 4.30pm, Shaun notices that Jennifer is unconscious. Her condition is serious and she is transferred to the intensive care unit. Fortunately, Jennifer makes a full recovery but her parents take legal action against the hospital for pain and suffering on the basis of dereliction of the duty of care to provide safe and timely treatment for Jennifer.

- What do you consider to be the main differences between the two situations?
- Do you consider there were mitigating circumstances for Shaun in not ensuring Jennifer's medication was administered?
- Do you think there are actions that Shaun could have taken to ensure appropriate and timely care could have been provided to all patients, including Jennifer?

Whatever your responses to questions two and three, it is very likely that you would agree that the two situations reflect different issues. In the first instance, the nurse has simply forgotten, and while we are all human, it would be reasonable to expect a registered nurse to administer prescribed treatment. The second example is not so clear cut. Clearly Shaun's ability to attend to Jennifer has been influenced by other demands within the ward environment. Whether or not these circumstances would represent a legally acceptable defence is difficult to determine; however, a number of issues would probably be considered, including:

- Should Shaun have contacted nursing administration with a request for more staff in response to the ward emergencies?
- Should Shaun have ensured that one staff member remained available to attend to the needs of other patients and ensure treatments were attended to as ordered?

The answers to questions such as these would determine whether or not Shaun had been derelict in his duty of care to Jennifer. That is, what would 'reasonably' be expected of a registered nurse in these circumstances?

Damage
This is relatively straightforward. Damage or injury must be evident if legal action for negligence is to be taken. If prescribed medication is not administered but the patient does not experience any ill-effects, there would be no basis for legal action.

Direct – cause and effect
The test that applies to determine causation is whether or not it 'is a reasonably foreseeable consequence of the defendant's negligent act' (Staunton & Chiarella, 2003: 36). This means it is not sufficient to show that damage or injury has occurred (in the case of Jennifer, unconsciousness), but this damage needs to have occurred as the result of the act or omission (failure to test blood glucose and administer insulin as prescribed).

The relationship between the cause (omission of treatment) and effect (unconsciousness) is likely to be seen as clear and obvious. However, it is important to note that Jennifer made a full medical recovery and legal action is based on pain and suffering, which is not so clearly obvious and would therefore be a matter of legal interpretation.

Policies and procedures

It is important that the distinction is made between laws on the one hand and policies and procedures on the other hand. Laws as discussed previously are enacted by state, territory or Commonwealth governments. Policies and procedures, on the other hand, are employer directives. For example, many Australian health services require that two nurses hear a telephone medication order before the medication can be given. This is a local rather than a legal requirement. The Drugs and Poisons Acts do not require this. In legal terms a court will give consideration to policies and procedures; however, if they disregard the law, are considered out of date, unobtainable or totally inappropriate the court can overrule them. Policies and procedures do not provide a defence for failure to adhere to legal expectations or responsibilities.

Example
A nurse working in a community mental health team is the only nurse on duty when an emergency phone order is required. Whilst the Drugs and Poisons Act states that only one nurse is required to hear the order the policies and

Continued

procedures of the health service state that two nurses are required for all phone orders. Legally the nurse is not prevented from taking the order; however, to do so would be breaching the health services policy.

Consider the two alternatives:

- If the nurse accepts the order he is breaching policy.
- If the nurse does not accept the order he could be found to have neglected his duty of care if damage or injury results.

If tested in a court of law the Drugs and Poisons Act for that jurisdiction would be considered as the definitive authority. Breaching the health service policy would be seen as necessary in that situation to avoid negligence.

The doctrine of vicarious liability

This concept originated from the master–servant relationship and describes the responsibility that the master had for the actions of his servants. In contemporary society it refers to the responsibility the employer holds for the actions of employees.

The basic assumption behind this concept is that the employer bears responsibility for the actions of employees where the employees operate within the bounds and expectations of their professional role. For nurses, this means that the hospital or health care organisation that employs them assumes the responsibility of providing safe and effective health care to the people who use its services.

The doctrine of vicarious liability imposes legal liability on a person or an organisation for another's wrong doing. In the case of the health care industry, the organisation may be found to be vicariously liable where:

(1) the tort or wrong doing was committed by a person as an employee
(2) the tort was committed during the time of employment.

However, there are limits to vicarious liability, particularly where employees knowingly operate outside their scope of practice. The organisation may take legal action against employees to claim damages paid or a proportion thereof when the employee's actions have diverted from what could reasonably be expected as part of their employment.

In terms of vicarious liability, as a rule:

- Organisations will support you if you have operated within your standards of practice.
- Operating outside the standards of practice could result in your organisation being sued by the person claiming compensation for your wrong doing.

- In turn the organisation may seek financial compensation from you.
- If you have breached policy, the insurance company representing the health service may sue you individually for compensation.
- Historically, nurses have not earned sufficient income for insurance companies to sue; however, that is changing as nurses now often have more assets, have higher incomes, etc.

Increasingly, professional indemnity insurance is advised to cover nursing practice. Professional indemnity may be included in the membership fees of professional and/or industrial bodies.

Reflective exercise

Check the conditions of membership of professional/industrial bodies of which you are either a member or eligible for membership:

- Do they provide professional indemnity cover?
- What amount are you covered for?
- Is that amount likely to be sufficient if a person becomes seriously injured or dies and the clinical supervision you have provided is considered to be a contributing factor?
- What are the conditions that exclude the insurance company from financial responsibility?
- Are there any provisions specifically made about clinical supervision?

Implications for clinical supervision

If clinical supervision is conducted according to the principles outlined in this book, it is unlikely that any adverse effect could be attributed to clinical supervision. As we have discussed in Chapter 1, the clinical supervisor does not (and should not) accept responsibility for the clinical practice of supervisees. Therefore, if a supervisee acts or fails to act in a manner that results in adverse outcomes, and this is claimed to have occurred as a direct result of the actions or advice of the clinical supervisor, this argument should be dismissed.

Legal action involving (either directly or indirectly) clinical supervision within nursing has not yet been witnessed in Australia. However, given the increased focus on clinical supervision for nurses it is possible that this may change in the future. If you agree to provide clinical supervision and something goes wrong you may be asked to demonstrate that you had the skills and appropriate preparation for the role and that you were not operating outside of your scope of practice. It is therefore crucial that you do not take on the role of clinical supervisor unless you feel confident and competent to do so. Education and training are essential as adequate preparation for this role and are discussed in further detail in Chapter 7.

Documenting clinical supervision

There is no legal obligation to keep process notes on clinical supervision sessions. However, we recommend that as a formal relationship, process notes are as important for clinical supervision as they are for health care and therapy.

Many people engaged in clinical supervision, particularly supervisees, do not feel comfortable about the idea of process notes. This usually reflects concern about confidentiality. It is important to remember that supervisors are likely to provide supervision for more than one person and it is therefore likely to be difficult to retain a comprehensive understanding of supervisees' issues and journeys without notes. Session notes are particularly useful in reviewing individual sessions and monitoring progress over time.

Confidentiality

While acknowledging the importance of process notes, confidentiality is likely to remain an issue of concern for many supervisees. There is likely to be concern that information about the supervisee's practice or other issues such as conflict with management or colleagues may become known to others outside of the supervisory relationship. This danger can be minimised through the way the notes are written. For example, the notes can refer to major themes rather than specific details and pseudonyms can be used in place of names.

Example

19.11.07 Notes of clinical supervision session with Mary Mathews
   Clinical scenario raised today by Mary – Major themes

- Altercation with a medical specialist (KP) in relation to the involvement of a patient and her family in treatment planning.
- The patient and family had expressed to Mary (primary nurse) that they did not feel heard or listened to and wanted her support in ensuring that their views were taken into consideration.
- Mary wanted to assist her patient but was feeling unsure about the best way to do this and wanted to explore her hesitation in some detail and problem solve the ways forward.
- Mary expressed she had experienced difficulty with KP in the past and she found it difficult to approach him due to this past experience.
- Mary also expressed she did not feel able to discuss this with her nurse unit manager (NUM) as she had not found her supportive when past issues about KP were raised.

Continued

Main discussions/overview

Through the exploration in supervision Mary identified that she was slightly intimidated by KP and found him to be dismissive of her and nurses in general. When Mary had tried to advocate for her patients in the past, Mary had found that KP was 'rude, abrupt and dismissive'. Mary discussed in some detail her own issues of authority and lack of assertion when it came to people in senior roles, e.g. NUMs, medical specialists, consultants and educators.

Mary identified that she needed to find ways to assert her patients' needs even when feeling intimidated by others. Throughout the rest of the supervision session we explored the reasons behind this and discussed ways for Mary to be able to feel more comfortable expressing and asserting herself, even when there might be a negative or direct response from her seniors. She developed a dialogue she felt comfortable with and she practiced saying this to KP and also to her NUM. Mary asked to role-play the interaction. Whilst this was the first time had Mary asked to use role-play, it seemed like a very useful strategy and she seemed to really use the medium well.

Mary left the session very confident in her ability to meet with KP the following day after ward round to discuss the patient and family's requests.

Need to check in next session as to the outcome.

Steps can be taken to protect the confidentiality of process notes, including the storage of notes in a locked filing cabinet which can only be accessed by the supervisor. This may alleviate some concerns of supervisees but it is also important that they have a realistic understanding of the limits of confidentiality. Confidentiality is not absolute and can be overridden by the public interest in the case of matters involving protection of the public and/or the prosecution of a serious crime. For example, if the death of a patient becomes a matter for the coroner's court, any documentation the court considers relevant can be ordered and must be provided. This would include process notes from clinical supervision if it was considered they may contribute to the investigation of cause of death.

Ownership and storage of process notes

There is no legal requirement to maintain notes in clinical supervision. However, issues of ownership are relevant if the notes are written in work time. In these circumstances, the records of clinical supervision from within an organisation are owned by the organisation. There is no specific legislation pertaining to clinical supervision records; as clinical information is very likely to be discussed they would be treated as a health care record (MacFarlane, 2000; Staunton & Chiarella, 2003), but you should refer to your state or territory's legal requirements for health records. However, generally the organisation owns the notes. In the case of private practice, the clinical supervisor has ownership over all documentation. As with all health records, correct storage is an essential requirement. However, you may need to refer to the relevant legislation. The information you obtain needs to be discussed with the supervisee, and the expectations of the organisation employing you need to be clearly understood.

You need to spend some time reflecting on the issue of process notes. For some supervisors this is not an easy clear-cut decision and there may be some homework involved prior to starting.

Questions to be asked

- Is there an expectation from my organisation that I keep notes?
- Who owns the clinical supervision notes?
- Who has access to the notes?
- Is a locked cabinet available?
- What will happen to the notes when the clinical supervision ends?

Legal jurisdictions of relevance to nurses

Nurses may appear at or face the following courts or hearings:

- professional body, e.g. nursing registration authority
- coroner's court
- civil court (magistrates' court)
- conciliation.

Nursing registration authority

The nursing registration authorities of the respective states and territories of Australia have a responsibility to ensure that professional standards of conduct are maintained. Anyone can report a nurse to the relevant nursing registration authority on the basis of unprofessional conduct or illegal behaviour. Nursing registration authorities have the power to sanction the behaviour or actions of nurses through the cancellation or suspension of registration.

Coroner's court

The role of the coroner's court is to investigate the cause of death. Unlike other courts, a person cannot be found innocent or guilty. The coroner can suggest that people have contributed to the cause of death through statements like 'the two nurses in this particular situation contributed to this person's death by . . . administering the wrong medication'. If the coroner has concerns that the level of contribution has implications for criminal law, he or she can refer the case with the cause of death to the public prosecutor's office. However, a more likely scenario is that the public prosecutor's office receives all coroners' reports and makes a decision on whether to prosecute independently.

Civil court (magistrates' court)

Magistrates' courts hear both criminal and civil cases. Only the police can prosecute under criminal law; however, private individuals can pursue civil action. Nurses may appear in civil cases as a defendant or be called in as an expert witness.

Ethical issues

What is ethics?

The term 'ethics' relates to a process of determining the moral virtue of a particular course of action. It provides the basis from which people can:

> '. . . question why they considered a particular act right or wrong, what the reasons (justifications) are for their judgements, and whether their judgements are correct'. (Johnstone, 2004: 11)

Ethical principles

Staunton & Chiarella (2003) describe five main ethical principles:

(1) Concern for the well-being of individuals and of society.
(2) Embodiment of ideals, that is 'what should be done' is valued over 'what can be done'. Eliminating world hunger, for example, represents an ethical stance, despite the numerous and significant barriers that mean this goal is unlikely to be achieved in the foreseeable future.
(3) Use moral reasoning to determine what is appropriate or inappropriate in specific situations.
(4) Ethical principles are applied universally and equally, to all persons at all times.
(5) Ethics is considered to be of ultimate importance, more so than the law or other influences such as politics. Ethical decisions should also prevail over individual interests. For example, those who believe in the right of individuals to die with dignity would consider assisting a person with a terminal illness to end their life to be ethically correct despite the fact that the law stipulates such a practice as illegal. Under these circumstances the individual would probably consider the law to be unethical.

An ethical dilemma occurs when you need to make a decision but you are unsure of the action you should take. For example, there may be conflict between what you know you should do and what you want to do. Or perhaps you have an apparent conflict between two sets of ethical principles or between the values you hold.

Ethical issues can affect nurses on either an individual or a professional basis. At an individual level, nurses are influenced by their own views of behaviour and actions that they consider to be right or wrong. At a professional level nurses are governed by a code of ethics. The Australian Nursing and Midwifery Council (ANMC) has developed a Code of Ethics for Australian Nurses. This document can be downloaded from the ANMC website at: http://www.anmc.org.au/docs/Publications/ANMC%20Ethics%20for%20web.pdf.

Primarily the aim of this document is to outline the importance and essential characteristics of safe and professional nursing practice.

Ethics and clinical supervision

No specific guidelines have as yet been developed in relation to clinical supervision. However, as nursing practice poses a number of ethical dilemmas it is important that this area is explored.

Due to the complexity of nursing ethics, this topic will be further explored with the use of four scenarios which address the following areas:

(1)   nurse–patient relationships
(2)   confidentiality
(3)   group supervision – dealing with bullying
(4)   providing clinical supervision internal to the organisation.

Scenario 1: Nurse–patient relationships

Shannon (supervisor) and Sally (supervisee) work in different areas of the same organisation. They have been working together in supervision for over 2 years and have a strong and productive supervisory relationship. Sally had been a community mental health nurse (case manager) for many years; she is an outgoing and popular team member who is considered by her manager and peers to be a sound clinician and a 'good nurse'. Sally enjoys supervision, finds it very useful and makes effective use of the supervision sessions. She always comes prepared with clinical situations, and is able to be open and honest with Shannon about her work.

Today's session, however, became a little more difficult for Sally when the supervisor discussed with Sally her 'connection to a patient called Shane'. Shannon highlighted that Sally talked a lot about Shane and seemed to focus on him in a different way from that of other patients. Sally was initially quite surprised by this and then somewhat reluctantly admitted that her manager had also discussed with her recently her professional boundaries in relation to Shane. She was, for example, spending considerable time with him, working back late, and having Shane as the last appointment of the day, etc. Sally admitted to

Shannon that she had not realised she was doing this, but it became obvious when the manager pointed it out.

Sally also admitted to Shannon that she had thought of bringing Shane to supervision (through the supervision process) a number of times as Shane reminded her of her ex-boyfriend and working with him had raised issues for her in relation to the break up with her ex-boyfriend. Sally also talked about how much she was really enjoying working with Shane; they were similar ages, he was not as unwell as her other clients and she gained much from their work together. Sally was not able to articulate why she had not discussed this within supervision previously.

When Shannon asked if Sally was attracted to Shane, Sally was clearly uncomfortable and quietly answered 'Yes'. Sally then very quickly stated that she knew it was not okay but had it under control, that she was professional and handling it well and also felt that she had hidden her 'secret' feelings from Shane. Sally seemed really embarrassed and talked about how she should be able to handle her feelings and not be attracted to a patient and not let it affect her work. Sally also seemed clear that until now Shane had had 'no idea' of her feelings. However, after their last session Shane had given Sally his telephone number and asked her to give him a call.

Sally admitted, again in an embarrassed and uncomfortable way, that, although she did not call him and they have not had contact since, she was struggling as part of her had really wanted to call.

Reflective exercise

(1) What are the ethical dilemmas in the above scenario?
(2) As the clinical supervisor explore each of these ethical dilemmas in detail in relation to the following:
 • What would I do next?
 • How would my organisation expect me to react?
 • How could I support Sally?
 • What supports (including administrative supports like policies/procedures) are available to support me in making these decisions?

Consider your answers to the questions above. How much of how you responded was based on fact and how much was influenced by what you think you know or what you think might have happened? It is absolutely essential in supervision that you only respond to what you are told, that you do not gap fill and assume or guess. For example, you know Sally is attracted to Shane, you know he gave her his telephone number and you know that part of her wanted to call.

In this scenario some supervisors may believe that Sally is already having an affair or disbelieve her and think she really did call him. You do not know that and to make up details based on your own imagination, bias and prejudices is dangerous.

Sally needs your support and understanding. Disclosing attraction to a patient is difficult and it would be really easy to shame Sally and make her feel like she is a 'bad nurse'. Supervisors need to put aside their own feelings of disgust, disbelief and frustration in circumstances such as these. Sally needs you to acknowledge that attractions can occur, that it is normal, at times, to be attracted to patients and the important thing is how we manage the attraction. Patients are human beings after all and attractions between humans are bound to occur at different times, even when they are not supposed to. As her supervisor, you would need to find a way to work with Sally to gently explore the issues around patient boundaries. Some of the questions you might pose to Sally include:

- What are professional boundaries?
- Why do we have clear boundaries between patients and staff?
- What are the consequences for the patient and staff if these boundaries are breached?
- Does Sally think that she has breached any boundaries at this stage?

Sally's response to these questions will depend on the way you as a supervisor continue to address this situation with her. If Sally continues to be clear that she is not to call, and that relationships with patients are not acceptable and she is able to articulate the reasons why, then you as her supervisor will be able to remain working with Sally in a fairly supportive and non-directive way. However, if Sally is unclear about professional boundaries and questions why she cannot go out with Shane, or states that she plans to call him, then you as Sally's supervisor would be likely to manage the rest of the session quite differently. You are not required to make your own subjective decision in this situation; it is not up to you as a supervisor to say whether a staff member can or cannot commence a relationship with a patient. That decision is made by professional registration bodies via codes of conduct statement/polices, organisational polices and even team-/ward-based guidelines. You as the supervisor need to use these ethical and legal frameworks to support and guide you in the work you do with Sally. You are not alone; you do not have to make these decisions alone.

In fact, you also may have identified other dilemmas or questions in this scenario for which there is no clear cut answer, for example:

- Should Shannon have raised the issue of Shane at all as supervision should be directed by the supervisee?

- Sally may become suspicious (rightly or wrongly) that the manager and supervisor had spoken together as both had raised the issue of Shane.
- How much of what Sally may raise in relation to Shane is appropriate to supervision and how much might need to be taken somewhere else? For example, unresolved issues about the break up with her boyfriend may be more appropriately explored in therapy rather than supervision.

These are all really good questions and there are no easy answers. Your explorations with Sally throughout the session will guide you and provide you with the direction you need to go in. Just remember to support Sally. This is a complex, difficult and very sensitive issue and Sally needs and deserves our support and understanding; she does not deserve to be shamed and humiliated. She also needs to feel comfortable in continuing to discuss the matter. If you show obvious signs of disapproval, Sally may stop raising the matter with you and therefore lose an opportunity for support and guidance as she works through the issue.

Scenario 2: Manager–supervisor relationships

Daniel is reading the paper in the tea room when Tricia, an NUM, enters and asks Daniel if he has a moment. Before waiting for a response Tricia loudly launches into a diatribe about her concern about a staff member on her ward named Jenny.

Tricia states she knows that Jenny sees Daniel for supervision and begins firing questions at Daniel about the supervision relationship and the supervision sessions. For example:

- Does Jenny use her supervision sessions?
- How do you think she is going?
- Have you noticed if anything is wrong with Jenny?
- Are you concerned in any way about her practice?
- What is she using clinical supervision for?

Tricia also states she has a number of concerns about Jenny and her performance and has had a number of complaints from other staff and patients about Jenny's behaviour and manner.

Daniel is clearly uncomfortable, caught off guard and taken aback by the manager and her questions. He is particularly taken aback by the intimidating way the manager is standing over him in a public place demanding a response to these questions.

Daniel asks the manager if she would like to sit down to chat about this further. He politely explains to Tricia that he is unable to discuss the contents of the supervision session as they are confidential.

Tricia is extremely dissatisfied with this reply and becomes increasingly more frustrated and visibly annoyed with Daniel. Tricia begins blaming everything on clinical supervision – she states that she understood that one of the reasons that the organisation was looking to implement supervision was to improve standards of care and to support managers and staff. Because of this she considers it reasonable that Daniel discuss Jenny's performance with her, especially if there are concerns.

When Daniel suggests the manager talks directly to Jenny and asks her how she is going, the manager raises her voice and states, 'I have spoken to Jenny, I have had her in my office on several occasions due to poor performance and complaints. I do not want to speak with Jenny, I want to speak with you as her clinical supervisor. I want to know from you as a senior member of staff in this program what is going on with *my* staff'. Tricia further expresses she is concerned she might have an incompetent staff member on her ward and that is far more serious that the 'breach of confidentiality' Daniel is hiding behind.

Tricia argues that as the manager it is unacceptable that she is 'kept out of the loop' and that clinical supervision was supposed to be about helping staff. Tricia also tells Daniel she released staff to attend supervision on the assumption that the outcomes would be favourable, but clearly it was not working as she had not seen an improvement in Jenny's performance. Whilst it was not said, there is a clear underlying threat that Tricia may remove her support for her nurses attending supervision.

Daniel then states he will talk to Jenny to seek her permission to discuss details of the supervision sessions. He hopes that Jenny would agree, but without her permission he cannot discuss the details. Daniel does state that Jenny uses the clinical supervision sessions well and always attends. Again Tricia is not happy with this suggestion and the interaction ends when the manager says she is going to be completing Jenny's appraisal in the next few weeks and will officially request Daniel's involvement.

Reflective exercise

(1) What are the ethical dilemmas in the above scenario?
(2) Do you think it is important for the clinical supervisor to keep the supervision sessions confidential and keep them focused on and driven by the supervisee?
(3) How do you feel about the way Daniel responded in this situation?
(4) Why is it important to keep managers engaged and supportive of clinical supervision? As the supervisor in the above scenario how might you do this?
(5) What would Daniel's responsibility be to the organisation if he had major concerns about Jenny's competence in supervision?

Continued

(6) What is the manager's responsibility if she was concerned about Jenny's competence? How does this relate to clinical supervision?

(7) What should Daniel do next in relation to the request/demand from the manager to be involved in the appraisal?

(8) What structures/systems should an organisation implement to reduce the likelihood of a situation like this occurring?

(9) How do you think you would respond in this situation? How vulnerable are you to managers standing over you? What if Tricia had been the opposite and politely approached you seeking your support as she was concerned for Jenny and felt that you might be able to assist her in working more effectively with Jenny and helping her out – how might you have responded in that situation?

In this scenario the most important skill is how the supervisor protects the supervisee whilst not totally alienating the manager. This is often easier said than done, particularly where the manager is being intimidating and threatening. This can often be complicated further if you are all in the same organisation and the manager and supervisor have a professional relationship outside of this discussion. Remember that while managers do not control what is in the supervision session they are instrumental in supporting the implementation of supervision and hence alienating them is not advisable. In fact, it could mean the end of clinical supervision for some or all staff in that team. Supervisors and managers must find a way to work together.

In the above scenario it was evident Tricia did not have a clear understanding of clinical supervision. She did not appear to be aware of the boundaries of supervision and the fact that clinical supervision and line management were two different functions undertaken by different people, in parallel, but in isolation from each other.

Daniel therefore needed to support and educate the manager while at all times protecting the integrity of the supervision with Jenny. This is best done by Daniel speaking in hypothetical and generalities rather than specifics. Within this education Daniel would also be able to educate the manager about the concept of clinical supervision and confidentiality and that it is not absolute. If Daniel had serious concerns, hypothetically if required he would have to support Jenny to talk to her manager. His role is to support Jenny and assist her to talk to management rather than him talking without Jenny's knowledge, but he also has certain responsibilities as a supervisor which he took seriously, just as Tricia did as the manager.

In the above scenario did you realise that Daniel actually got caught out in the end? He actually agreed to take the manager's concerns to supervision and ask Jenny if she was happy with him talking to her manager. Daniel allowed Tricia's agenda to invade Jenny's supervision. How do you think Jenny might respond? Understandably, she is likely to be distressed that her supervisor and manager are talking and perhaps even be fearful or concerned her confidentiality has not been respected. By bringing in the manager's agenda Daniel was not respecting Jenny's right to drive the supervision sessions.

This is clearly a difficult situation for Daniel but it is a not uncommon one in supervision. Organisations need to ensure that they implement clinical supervision in an informed and respectful way to protect the supervision process and ensure managers are also clear about what supervision is and is not, and how they can gain support for what is often a very challenging role. This also signifies the importance of written policies, which can serve as a useful reference point for supervisors to be able to clarify clinical supervision and its associated boundaries.

Scenario 3: Bullying raised in group supervision

Rachel has been providing clinical supervision for an inpatient medical team for 14 months. She works in a different department of the same organisation. During this period there have been a number of changes occurring within the workplace, and some conflict has emerged between team members. There has been a stable core group of nurses attending supervision on a regular basis. However, in the last 3 weeks the group have been unusually quiet, the conversation has not flowed. This session started off in much the same way, then a couple of staff encouraged others to talk and one started to cry.

Sandra starts to talk about how intimidated they feel at work because of the behaviour and attitudes of some staff members. This has got to the point that they do not want to come to work when these people are on duty. The manager does not know what is happening because they are too scared to tell him; they think this will only make things worse. Sick leave is on the rise and one staff member is planning to leave.

They describe frequently feeling humiliated in front of their peers. Rachel is concerned about the level of distress in the room and the significance of the bullying being described. The nurses feel undermined and set up. They feel the workload is not evenly distributed and some people just are not able to get through what they are given.

Rachel asks them whether they have spoken to the person concerned about his behaviour and the impact of this upon them. They indicated that one person had tried but she had been yelled at. The others did not wish to experience the same behaviour so they attempted to stay away from him as much as possible.

Reflective exercise

(1) What are the ethical dilemmas in the above scenario? Explore them in detail.
(2) How should the clinical supervisor start to explore these issues?
(3) Can you identify any complicating factors in this situation?
(4) Would the situation be different in any way if the clinical supervisor was external to the organisation?
(5) How could the clinical supervision be structured within the organisation to support Rachel managing this situation, that is who can supervise whom?
(6) Would you manage things differently in a group supervision session rather than in an individual session? If so, in what ways?
(7) What are the policies on bullying in your organisation?

It is important to keep in mind that people can often feel quite power-less in the face of bullying. They may not attempt to seek help, instead choosing sick leave or resignation. As the clinical supervisor you walk the line of listening and being supportive but not further undermining an individual's difficulty in coping by reinforcing the inability to manage the situation. The supervisor's role is to help individuals understand what the organisational structures are that may support them and help them to explore their options, providing time to develop an understanding of the consequences of the choices available. Clinical supervisors are valuable to their supervisees primarily by assisting them to explore how they might address specific issues.

For example, if you were the clinical supervisor in this example you might want to explore the perception that 'speaking with the manager will make things worse'. What is the evidence that this is the case? How do they imagine the situation would become worse?

It is very important that you are aware of what is being evoked in yourself. You may have experienced some bullying in the past and you must be able to separate your own experience from that of the super-visees. It would be problematic for all concerned if you started to direct them to a course of action that represented what you would have liked for yourself rather than what is in the best interest of the supervisees.

People need to feel supported but also to consider what they and the environment they work in contribute to the situation. For example, a nurse who is new to the role of ANUM is being accused of bullying. When the situation is investigated it appears this nurse received little, if any, orientation to the role, which suggests a lack of organisational support. The nurse is quite stressed by a lack of understanding of the role and this is expressed by being curt and snappy with other staff.

It is important to keep in mind some of the issues that are central to providing group supervision. The response to the questions you pose and how you respond to the distress of individual group members will be magnified for the individual by the fact that it happens in front of colleagues. It may be useful to summarise at the end or encourage someone from the group to do this. This provides you with an opportunity to hear back how the discussion has been understood. You do not want to alienate people. They need to be heard but you also do not want to lose your capacity to support them through the dilemma.

You may also come under pressure to rescue group members from the situation. For example, you might offer to take an issue to the manager yourself. As an internal supervisor you are more vulnerable to these types of boundary pressures and if you have a tendency to want to rescue people or actively solve their problems (characteristics that are not uncommon for nurses) you will need to maintain your awareness of this tendency and ensure you keep it in check. It is important not to foster dependence on the supervisor or convey the message that supervisors can manage situations more effectively than supervisees.

Scenario 4: Sonya supervising within her organisation
Sonya has been working for 10 years in her current organisation; she is well known and respected by her colleagues and by management. As a result Sonya is often chosen by her peers as a clinical supervisor. Management support Sonya in this role because they recognise her as providing valuable support for her colleagues.

Sonya is supervising Kate, a nurse working in a surgical unit. She is currently undertaking her graduate year. Sonya and Kate have been working together in supervision since Kate commenced. Kate has been an enthusiastic supervisee; she has attended regularly and taken responsibility for bringing issues to discuss. In recent sessions Kate has raised concerns about her relationship with her colleagues. She has been feeling like people are not happy with her and she is not sure what the problem is. She said that she has trouble with one of the senior staff who tends to be very directive, always telling her what to do. She acknowledges that she has an entirely different style and occasionally she thinks that it is a problem but finds the constant direction hard. Kate realises that there are many ways to do things but feels they always have to be done the way this person wants it; she does not allow for any difference. Kate describes times when she has done things her way rather than the way she was told to but the outcome was the same positive outcome. Kate's concern about working with this senior staff member is that she will not learn how to think for herself or trust her own abilities. She does not want to have to rely on being directed to do something all the time.

Sonya knows Kate's manager and although they are working in different teams their paths do cross in some meetings. Sonya finds herself in the situation of hearing the manager debriefing about managing a staff member (Kate). She found out in the meeting that it was another staff member who had reported Kate and there is a very large difference in the stories relayed. In general, there has not been any issue of concern for Sonya in her role as clinical supervisor until this moment when she learns that Kate was about to be given a warning and she finds herself in a very awkward place.

Sonya does not participate in the discussion but feels very uncomfortable and excuses herself, but she has already heard more than she is comfortable with. She has a clinical supervision session with Kate that afternoon and is very uncomfortable knowing what she does.

When Kate comes to the session she reports that the situation has improved and the senior staff member has backed off and is letting her do things her way now and she is feeling better about working with them.

Reflective exercise

(1) What are the ethical dilemmas in the above scenario? Explore them in detail.
(2) How should the clinical supervisor respond to Kate in this situation?
(3) What are the complicating factors in this situation?
(4) What is the impact of the clinical supervisor being from the same organisation rather than external?
(5) How could the clinical supervision be set up within the organisation to support Sonya managing this situation?
(6) What should Sonya's response to the manager be if any?

This scenario serves as a reminder of the need for supervisors of having their own clinical supervision to assist them to manage their feelings about being a supervisor and dealing with the inherent stressors involved. This scenario represents a possible stressor. It is the supervisee who determines the content of the session not the supervisor. As a clinical supervisor it is not your role to introduce information you hear about them or other colleagues into the sessions. As difficult as it is to be privy to this sort of information, it may be necessary to remind managers and staff broadly via the supervision coordinator of the importance of being mindful of supervisory relationships and not having conversations in front of staff that would result in placing them in the difficult position of having information about a supervisee that could potentially compromise that relationship.

As the supervisor, you may be tempted to tell Kate what you know. However, doing so would raise a range of potential implications that would be problematic. Indeed, the supervisee may become more anxious or distressed and not know how to deal with this information. Kate may confront the manager and further fuel the conflict. It is important to ask yourself why you would consider saying anything. Is it to make yourself feel better because you do not have to hold information that is uncomfortable? This is understandable but is not a reasonable justification to take this type of action.

Mandatory vs voluntary clinical supervision

The key to addressing this issue may well lie in considering the fact that it is difficult and maybe even impossible to mandate a successful relationship. People may be forced to sit in a room together but you cannot make them talk about their work in a meaningful way. It is, however, frustrating for some that the people believed to be most in need of clinical supervision are often those who do not want it. It is understandable that this may be an issue of concern; however, it is important to consider why we may think this way and what it says about our views or understanding of clinical supervision. If by 'those who most need it' we refer to 'problem' staff, this suggests that a primary aim of clinical supervision is to work with staff who are not functioning well, almost as a form of remedial action, rather than promoting a relationship aimed at increasing understanding of and working towards the improvement of clinical practice.

Clinical supervision is therefore needed by everyone. All staff should be accessing the support they need to work as effectively and confidently as possible. This may lead to the conclusion that it should be mandatory. However, again it is important to consider how effective force or coercion is likely to be. Some organisations have dealt with this issue by describing clinical supervision as an expectation. This terminology reflects the idea that supervision is important and supported by management but falls short of insisting that it happens.

The choice of supervisor is also an important consideration. Sometimes nurses are allocated to specific supervisors. This can present a deterrent, particularly to those who are already a bit reluctant. The more people are involved in the process the more they are likely to value it and commit to it. Choosing one's supervisor is an important part of feeling involved.

Clinical supervision is a responsible role that should be taken on with consideration given to the environment that it will be conducted in and what the supports are that will enhance success. It should not be entered into lightly. As you will have seen from this chapter there are a number of complex issues that can be raised, and a clinical supervisor needs to be adequately prepared and supported to function well in the role.

Conclusion

As a profession nursing must be cognisant of the broader legal and ethical implications associated with practice and health care. Clinical supervision as a part of professional practice is influenced by legal requirements and ethical considerations. Given the absence of the legal regulation of clinical supervision, it is important that the broader expectations are considered. In this chapter, the potential legal implications of clinical supervision have been discussed. Ethical issues that may arise have also been described and considered by the use of scenarios representing situations that may occur in practice. The issue of whether clinical supervision should be mandatory or voluntary has also been examined.

References

Johnstone, M.J. (2004) *Bioethics: A Nursing Perspective.* (4th edn). Sydney: Churchill Livingstone.

MacFarlane, P. (2000) *HEALTH LAW Commentary & Materials.* Annadale NSW: The Federation Press.

Staunton, P.J. & Chiarella, M. (2003) *Nursing and the Law.* (5th edn). Marrickville, NSW: Elsevier.

Enhancing the supervisory relationship: the roles of the supervisor and supervisee

Introduction

Successful clinical supervision occurs as a direct result of the quality of the relationship between supervisor and supervisee. Achieving a quality relationship is heavily reliant on the skill and expertise of the supervisor. The supervisor assumes an important and responsible role, and therefore must receive appropriate theoretical and practical preparation. Supervisors also have an obligation to ensure that they practice safely and correctly.

The role of supervisee is also crucial to achieving productive outcomes. If the primary importance of clinical supervision is to enhance nursing practice through reflection and professional development, it is crucial that supervisees receive guidance to obtain the maximum benefit from supervision. However, the role of supervisee is certainly not a passive one. On the contrary, supervisees also need skills and knowledge in order to make effective use of clinical supervision.

The aim of this chapter is to explore the roles of clinical supervisor and supervisee, and consider the factors that must be achieved in order to strengthen these roles and therefore enhance the supervisory relationship. More specifically the contents of this chapter include:

- skills and knowledge required to provide supervision
- what the supervisor needs to know about the supervisee
- the importance of education and training
- supervisor burnout, what it is and how to avoid it
- establishing boundaries for safe practice
- the importance of self-awareness and reflection
- choosing the right supervisor for you
- what the supervisee needs to know about the supervisor

- making the most of clinical supervision
- education and training for supervisees
- dealing with issues that may arise in the supervisory relationship.

The clinical supervisor

Skills and knowledge to provide supervision

Becoming a clinical supervisor is a responsible senior position and clinicians need to be sure they are prepared for that responsibility. It is likely that managers will have an active role in identifying suitable staff and encouraging them to take on this role. However, it is very important that nurses agree to become clinical supervisors without pressure or coercion. Nurses who are persuaded or forced into this role are unlikely to approach the role with the level of commitment required to ensure successful outcomes.

Reflective exercise

Consider the following questions:

- Do you want to be a clinical supervisor?
- Why would you choose to become a clinical supervisor?
- What are your motivations and what do you hope you achieve from providing clinical supervision?
- Do you have the support of your organisation to become a clinical supervisor?

If your answers suggest that you feel forced or pressured into becoming a clinical supervisor by your organisation and that your heart is not really in it or you feel under-prepared then you have a responsibility to discuss this with someone. There may be some tough decisions you have to make about whether you are willing to take on the responsibility of becoming a clinical supervisor. It is a big responsibility for you but something you owe to future supervisees.

Supervisors need to be qualified senior staff with experience of clinical supervision. This experience should come from formal education and training, and also from their own personal experience as a supervisee. It is important to clarify and seek a common understanding of what is meant by 'senior' staff. Within organisations, seniority is often defined according to one's position within the hierarchy. This may be reinforced by including the expectation that nurses in higher level positions provide clinical supervision and the inclusion of this as a criterion on position descriptions.

This expectation does not take into consideration whether someone is qualified and prepared to provide supervision. Defining seniority in such a narrow way also negates the view of clinical seniority. Some nurses choose not to apply for promotions because they prefer to remain closer to the clinical environment. In a clinical sense these nurses may be very senior even if they are not at a high level in the nursing hierarchy. Furthermore, they often have a wealth of experience to offer as a clinical supervisor. To overlook these nurses because of their position within the hierarchy could result in the waste of a potentially valuable resource.

Defining seniority through years of experience can also be problematic. While years of experience can be valuable, this is not the same as expertise, which is gained through the active development of skill and knowledge according to the principles of life-long learning. It is likely we have all worked with nurses who have been in a role for a lengthy period but tend to just go through the motions without reflecting and continuing to learn and develop. On the other hand, we can probably all identify nurses with considerably less experience who approach the job with passion and enthusiasm, continually seeking opportunities to learn new information in order to improve practice and patient care. As will become apparent throughout this chapter, these characteristics are far more important than the amount of time spent in nursing.

When clarifying the characteristics of a good or effective clinical supervisor it is useful to divide them into two main categories: interpersonal skills and practical skills.

Interpersonal skills

Interpersonal skills are those that make us human and are often those skills that are essential for nurses in order to care for their patients. While some of the skills can be taught and are in some ways quite practical, they are often more easily defined as personality traits. Some examples of 'good' interpersonal skills in a supervisor include being non-judgemental, open and honest, warm, friendly, engaging, having a good sense of humour, being insightful and self-reflective, and the ability to gently and respectfully challenge or question people without seeming critical. Furthermore, he or she must be authentic and have a genuine interest in becoming a clinical supervisor.

Practical skills

A clinical supervisor needs to be highly skilled as a communicator. This includes the ability to actively listen, ask clarifying questions and summarise the main points or issues. It is also important that clinical supervisors have sound clinical skills and are respected within the organisation, or have what is commonly termed as 'street cred'. This is where the different perspectives of management and clinicians may be in conflict. For example, managers may tend to place a high value on nurses who are able to practice efficiently and safely or who are reliable and punctual. Clinicians may be more concerned about clinical skills and the ability to communicate with patients and other nurses. As clinicians are the target population for clinical supervision it is advantageous to involve them in the process of identifying suitable supervisors, for example by nominating nurses they believe would make suitable supervisors (see Chapter 3).

The model of supervision the clinical supervisor uses is also very important. Clinical supervisors need to be able to articulate the model(s) or style(s) of clinical supervision they use in order to help supervisees select a suitable person to undertake supervision with. Although some supervisors may subscribe to a specific model, there are many who are influenced by a range of ideas and concepts through a combination of formal education and clinical experience. They are also likely to be influenced by the style of their own clinical supervisors. Whatever the model and whatever the style it is essential to be able to articulate it. Nurses have been traditionally less comfortable than other health professionals in being able to do this and will often describe themselves as eclectic. Eclectic is fine, many nurses practice in a holistic way; however, more detail is needed in what way are you eclectic, what models do you draw from, how do you structure your clinical supervision sessions?

Reflective exercise

Consider the skills you have that would assist you in the role of clinical supervisor. In particular think about:

- How would you describe yourself?
- How do you think others would describe you? What would they say are your strengths and areas that may require further development:
  - friends
  - family
  - patients
  - colleagues
  - managers?
- Imagine you are asked to describe yourself to someone who does not know you. What would you say?
- What are some of your interpersonal skills and what are some of the practical skills you have that would assist you as a clinical supervisor?
- What do you think a supervisee needs to know about you?

Reflective exercise

Now that you have thought a bit more about yourself, and your skills and ability, it is time to write an introduction to promote yourself as a potential supervisor. This does not have to be long and can be written in a variety of ways (formal CV style, creative and fun like an advertisement, a few formal or informal paragraphs that provide a comprehensive overview). How you structure this 'advertisement' says something about you . . .

The following hints may help you to decide what to include:

- area of clinical specialty
- clinical experience
- education and training in clinical supervision
- experience as a supervisor
- supervision model and/or style
- own supervision experience
- human attributes.

Reflective exercise

When you have completed the promotional blurb ask some colleagues you trust to review what you have written about yourself and comment on it. It is quite possible they will have a lot to add. As people and as nurses we often tend to understate our skills, knowledge and qualities. Now rewrite your promotional blurb based on this feedback. How does it look now? Would this adequately describe you as a clinical supervisor to someone who does not know you?

Being prepared and able to provide high-quality supervision also requires supervisors to have knowledge about supervisees. In this section, you are encouraged to consider the sorts of things that supervisees might want to know about you.

Reflective exercise

Consider the information you would like about potential supervisees in order to decide if the supervisory relationship is likely to be productive and successful. If you are receiving supervision or have done so previously you can probably answer this from your own personal experience.

Some ideas that you might want to include are presented in Table 7.1.

Table 7.1 What supervisors want to know about supervisees.

(1) Professional characteristics
(2) Experiences of supervision
(3) Motivation for seeking clinical supervision
(4) Expectations of clinical supervision and the clinical supervisor
(5) Preferred learning style

(1) Professional characteristics

It is important to allow your supervisees to introduce themselves to you. We can sometimes make the assumption, particularly if we work in the same organisation, that we know each other well. It is essential not to make the assumption that you know the person coming to supervision. Let supervisees talk about their professional life, their discipline and area of specialty, their education and training, including professional qualifications. There are a couple of reasons for this: firstly, you can learn a lot about the person sitting opposite, and secondly, and most importantly, you will be able to ascertain the qualifications and skills of the supervisees so that in clinical supervision you have an understanding of whether they are operating within their scope of practice and their skills set when they present clinical scenarios.

For example, a nurse working in oncology may inform you that he has completed advance training in cannulation and providing chemotherapy (cytotoxic medications). If he then describes a clinical scenario in which he describes being involved in the administration of chemotherapy you will feel comfortable that that is appropriate.

Ask supervisees to talk about themselves in depth as a clinician, their strengths, what they feel confident with. Ask them to describe their struggles or challenges as a clinician, and identify the areas where further development is needed.

(2) Experiences of supervision

In particular, it is important to know more about supervisees' attitudes, expectations and goals around clinical supervision. The following questions might help to elicit this information:

- Have you ever had clinical supervision before?
- If so, what was your experience of it?
- If not, what have you heard about clinical supervision and what do you think it is?

These questions are very important. If the supervisee has accessed supervision before and had a very negative experience it is quite likely that his or her attitude towards supervision will be a negative one. This needs to be discussed so that it can be worked through and also raises questions about why he or she is even accessing clinical supervision again. Similarly, if the supervisee has not had previous experience but heard only 'bad things' from those who have, he or she will probably be quite resistive.

The supervisee may have had a very positive experience of clinical supervision but had to choose another supervisor because the previous supervisor is no longer available. Supervisees may also seek supervision in response to positive feedback. While this can be encouraging, it may lead to unrealistic expectations of the supervisor and what clinical supervision can achieve.

Example 1

Theresa has worked for the same organisation since graduating 3 years ago. After hearing what clinical supervision 'is all about', she quickly expressed her interest. Theresa has been working in the paediatrics unit, which she loves, but feels she needs to learn more about family dynamics and how they impact on a child's recovery. She has chosen you as her supervisor because after some research she feels that you have valuable skills and knowledge she could learn from.

Example 2

Andrew is a registered nurse who is new to this organisation. Andrew has never had clinical supervision before, but has been told by his work mates that it is 'nothing more than a gripe session', that supervisors encourage you to talk about relationships within the organisation and then take it back to line managers. He has been warned not to believe all that stuff about privacy and confidentiality, but that what he says will find its way 'back to the bosses'.

Reflective exercise

Consider the two examples presented:

- What different challenges/opportunities do the two situations present?
- How important do you think the differences in attitudes would be for establishing a supervisory relationship?
- What strategies might you use to deal with Andrew's negative attitude?

(3) Motivation for seeking clinical supervision

Understanding why the supervisee has sought clinical supervision is an important step in establishing the relationship. It may be a workplace requirement rather than a matter of choice. Supervisees might consider that supervision will solve workplace problems, that they will be told how to do things better or that a magic solution to a specific problem will be easily found.

Asking the following questions might assist in gathering this information:

- Are you accessing supervision of your own free will or have you been pressured to do so? If you have been pressured, how does this make you feel about clinical supervision?
- Why now? Why are you seeking clinical supervision now?
- What do you hope or expect to gain from it?

If the supervisee has been coerced or pressured into engaging in supervision she or he is also likely to be resistive. While it is not your responsibility as a supervisor to engender enthusiasm, it is important to know the base you are starting from. If a supervisee has chosen or agreed to be involved in supervision they are likely to have goals and expectations, and probably an optimistic or at least curious attitude about what clinical supervision can achieve for them. If they have been coerced they will probably consider it at best a waste of time, and at worst a form of punishment.

(4) Expectations of clinical supervision and the clinical supervisor

The following is an example of some questions you might ask of a supervisee in order to begin your relationship with as clear an understanding as possible of what the supervisee expects from clinical supervision in general and from you in particular:

- Why have you chosen me as your supervisor? What particular skills or attributes do you identify in me? And how do you think they can be of value to you?
- What do you expect from clinical supervision?
- How do you think your practice might be influenced through participating in clinical supervision?
- How do you envisage yourself professionally at the end of 12 months? 5 years? 10 years? How do you feel that clinical supervision might contribute to your preferred future?

Reflective exercise

Consider and list any other factors you would like to know about your supervisee.

Discuss this idea with experienced supervisors. What questions do they ask of a new supervisee?

(5) Preferred learning style

People do not all learn in the same way. Common ways of learning include:

- visual – learn by seeing (reading, TV, photos, whiteboard), use words like 'see'.
- kinesthetic – learn by doing (games, warm-ups, practice sessions, note-taking).
- auditory – learn by listening (talking, sound, lectures, questions and answers).

People are generally capable of learning in a number of different ways; however, they usually have a preferred approach. Knowing how your supervisee likes to learn will assist you in knowing how to structure the sessions to ensure the supervisee gets the most out of them. Most people think of supervision as being two people sitting in an office spending an hour talking about a clinical issue. Supervision is thought of as something verbal, but this narrow view of supervision means that the supervisor is not adjusting the style to suit supervisees. For example, for a supervisee who identifies with you that they learn best by visual clues, sitting in a clinical supervision session for an hour talking is not going to be the most conducive learning environment for them. There will be much of the session they do not absorb or 'take in'. As a supervisor this is not being responsive to the supervisee's needs. For a visual supervisee a supervisor needs to utilise visual learning methods, such as butchers' paper, whiteboards, diagrams, watching or observing scenarios.

For a supervisee who learns by kinesthetics the supervisor needs to consider how to make the sessions more active, with warm-up exercises, practice sessions and role-plays, actively talking or working through sessions. To just sit and talk with a supervisee who learns best by doing again means that much potential for enhanced learning is missed.

To be able to respond to the differing needs of the supervisee is quite a challenge and the supervisor may need to consider whether or not he or she can provide supervision to everyone. For example, the supervisee may learn best by the use of practice sessions and role-plays, if you as a supervisor do not feel at all comfortable with this medium then you may not be the right supervisor for this supervisee.

Don't forget the supervisee

Supervisees should also be given the opportunity to ask any questions. It is important at this early stage to foster an environment of open communication so that the maximum value can be realised from the supervisory relationship.

Rights and responsibilities of a clinical supervisor

We often focus on the rights of the supervisee and forget that supervisors also have rights within the supervisory relationship. Along with rights there are also certain responsibilities.

An overview of the rights and responsibilities of clinical supervisors is presented in Table 7.2, adapted from Bond & Holland (1998: 86).

Table 7.2   Rights and responsibilities of clinical supervisors.

Rights	Responsibilities
As a supervisor you have the right to:	As a supervisor you have the responsibility to:
• be treated with respect as an equal partner in the supervision relationship • not be blamed for the shortcomings of the supervisees or the organisation • break confidentiality in exceptional circumstances as discussed in the clinical supervision agreement (see Chapter 8) • challenge behaviours, actions or statements from supervisees that cause you concern about their practice development or use of clinical supervision • challenge any statements or behaviours which are insulting or personally hurtful to you • refuse requests that make inappropriate demands on you in your role as clinical supervisor • be able to provide clinical supervision without outside interference from the supervisee's colleagues or manager or inappropriate requests from the supervisee • set personal and professional boundaries on what issues you are prepared to work on with the supervisee • choose whether or not to be a clinical supervisor for a particular person • take steps to withdraw from the clinical supervision relationship if you have difficulties in meeting the commitment or there are relationship difficulties that cannot be resolved.	• prepare for the clinical supervision session to ensure that there are no interruptions • revise notes from previous sessions • be reliable, adhering to agreed appointments, time boundaries, clinical supervision contract • maintain confidentiality except for exceptions as addressed in the clinical supervision agreement (see Chapter 8) • avoid raising any management or assessment issues • ensure that the session time is purely devoted to the clinical supervision contract and deal with other roles (if required) at other times • rebut inappropriate demands or outside interference from the supervisee's colleagues or manager or the supervisee trying to seek information from confidential supervision sessions • offer first-aid counselling, not psychotherapy for current burning issues but focus on how quality professional practice can be sustained in spite of personal difficulties • encourage the supervisee to seek specialist help or advice when necessary and to have access to sources of such help • challenge any behaviour or values which the supervisee displays or talks about which give you concern about their practice, development or use of clinical supervision • ensure that you yourself have the necessary back-up support, e.g. your own clinical supervision and support systems.

Ensuring the skills and competence of clinical supervisors

Despite the importance and value of the clinical supervision role, there is currently no established process for the regulation of clinical supervisors by nurse registration bodies. The state and territory governments of Australia have thus far provided little leadership in this area. The guidelines developed by the Department of Human Services, Victoria (2006) do not adequately address the issues of preparation and competency, clearly devolving this responsibility to individual mental health services.

The Department of Health, Western Australia (2005) developed a much more comprehensive guide with some direction and standards to support the implementation and sustainability of clinical supervision for nurses. However, the issue of competency was addressed only very briefly, with the expectation that the clinical supervisor:

- is a person trained/experienced with clinical supervision and should have a **minimum** of 2 years' experience in the mental health field
- is preferably from the same professional group
- is from the same or another worksite
- can give feedback at the supervisee's level of experience
- has at least the same or higher level of practice skills in the areas being addressed, but this is not absolutely necessary (p. 1).

Some of these issues, such as whether or not clinical supervision should be discipline specific, are a matter of debate and we have addressed these elsewhere (see Chapter 4). While it is important that consideration of the needs for skill and competence has been made, these criteria are quite general and neither individually nor in combination would they necessarily convince anyone that a clinical supervisor is adequately prepared and competent for the role. Individual organisations may have developed their own system for ensuring competency and it would be advised to inquire whether or not your organisation has a process in place.

The Western Australia guidelines are therefore a useful beginning point, but before we can be confident of the competence of clinical supervisors, the following criteria need to be met:

- The completion of appropriate education and training.
- Demonstration and maintenance of skills.
- Actively engaging in own supervision.

These three areas will be considered in further detail. However, this is not intended as a definitive or exhaustive list. Many factors influence the extent to which people consider themselves to be competent – you may think of others.

Reflective exercise

- To what extent do you consider yourself to be competent as a clinical supervisor?
- In what specific areas would you consider yourself to be competent?
- How have you determined that you are competent?
- How do you think you would be able to maintain competency in clinical supervision over time?

Education and training

Providing clinical supervision is a role with responsibility that should not be taken lightly or without some thought and preparation. Participation in a formal education or training program assists potential supervisors to develop understanding, skills and knowledge in this important role.

Until quite recently it was very difficult to find a training program for clinical supervision. The skills of clinical supervision were generally learned through experience. Often former clinical supervisors became role models. Learning from former clinical supervisors is an important and valid way to learn, in the same way as we tend to learn a great deal from other nurses we have worked with over the years. However, this form of learning is very much contingent on the skill of the clinical supervisor. Competent and effective clinical supervisors are excellent role models likely to influence the development of constructive skills and knowledge. The converse is also true, so that where the standards and practices of clinical supervisors are less than desirable, this is likely to influence the way their supervisees will operate when they provide clinical supervision to others.

Even where the clinical supervisor is skilled, knowledgeable and competent, he or she is an individual who has developed a style based on multiple factors such as experience, knowledge and personality. The supervisor will have an approach that has probably been developed over a period of time and has in effect become his or her style. Should the supervisee attempt to translate this approach into his or her own practice, the outcomes are likely to be problematic. Clinical supervisors need to learn and develop their own style, with learning from experience being just one potential learning area.

Furthermore, as acknowledged by the nursing profession through radical changes to its approach to education, a primary focus on learning by doing has its disadvantages. The main focus of supervision from the supervisee's perspective is related to clinical practice rather than to becoming a clinical supervisor. It is unlikely that the supervisee will be taken through a methodical learning process, covering a range of important issues that are built on one another and work towards the development of a solid skill set.

The importance of education and training has been acknowledged in the literature (McKeown, 2001; Clifton, 2002; Hancox *et al.*, 2004). Nurses do not have a long history and culture of supervision, and for many it is a new phenomenon. Their ability to learn from experience is therefore limited. However, it is not just the availability but also the quality of education and training that require careful consideration. There is considerable variation in the quantity and quality of available education (McKeown, 2001; Clifton, 2002; Hancox *et al.*, 2004).

In the absence of clear direction to guide the implementation of clinical supervision a range of education and training courses have been developed without any clear standards or even recommendations about the length or content of these courses. To the uninitiated, deciding which course is most suitable can be overwhelming. It is likely that the specific needs of individuals or organisations will influence the decision. However, certain considerations might help in choosing a course of suitable quality that is likely to meet organisational and/or individual needs. The following questions may provide a useful guide for this process:

- How long is the course? What objectives are expected to be achieved in the time frame? Length of time is not everything; however, courses of 1–2 days should be viewed with caution. Given the responsible and complex role of clinical supervision, and in order to adequately prepare the nurse for the role, it is inconceivable that it could be taught in less than 3 or 4 days.
- What is the content? The development of knowledge and skill is likely to be the primary focus of the training program. However, it is important that aspiring clinical supervisors attain a thorough and comprehensive understanding of clinical supervision and the many factors that influence its likelihood of success. Content should include:
  - understanding clinical supervision as distinct from other supervisory and clinical roles
  - the importance of clinical supervision for nursing and client care
  - the need for systematic implementation of clinical supervision
  - approaches to clinical supervision
  - models of clinical supervision
  - legal and ethical issues
  - skills and knowledge for the effective clinical supervisor
  - skills and knowledge for the effective clinical supervisee
  - the evaluation of clinical supervision.
- What teaching/learning approaches are used? Courses that mainly rely on didactic teaching approaches are likely to be limited in their

effectiveness. The success of clinical supervision is embedded in skill development. The most effective way to develop skills is through knowledge, experience and practice, translating theory into practice. Therefore, courses that also utilise experimental techniques such as role-plays/practice sessions are more likely to convey a realistic view of clinical supervision.

* How flexible is the content? Every organisation is different and is influenced by its own set of issues and dynamics. A one size fits all approach to course delivery is not likely to meet the specific needs of all organisations. An effective course needs to reflect this degree of flexibility. Better still, the course should provide the opportunity for prior consultation with key stakeholders from the organisation to ensure that the content is specifically designed to meet local needs. This would include an analysis of the organisation prior to training in order to establish specific needs and, if required, tailor part of the program to meet the organisation's needs.
* Is the course taught internally or externally? The implementation of clinical supervision as described in Chapter 3 highlights the importance of this debate. The primary advantage of education provided internally is largely economic. However, the importance of knowledge of the local context and the imperatives that are likely to influence the implementation of clinical supervision are also important. The primary advantage of external supervision is that it provides a degree of objectivity because the trainers are not employed by, and therefore do not have an investment in, the broader organisation. Referring back to Chapter 3, you will note that this level of detachment can be viewed as a significant advantage, particularly where there is low morale and cynicism about the motives of management. A combination of internal and external trainers has been posed as an approach that might capitalise on the positive aspects of both approaches.

Demonstrating competency

Education and training may be an important part of developing competency but on their own they are likely to be insufficient to ensure competency is both achieved and maintained. Engaging in one's own clinical supervision is an important part of maintaining the quality of the supervision (discussed below). Organisations that support and endorse clinical supervision for nurses and other health professionals have a responsibility to ensure that those professionals entrusted in this role have the skill and competency to carry it out. It is therefore important that processes are developed and enacted to ensure this is the case. Refresher courses and journal clubs, for example, can assist clinical supervisors to remain current and competent.

Reflective exercise

- What other initiatives might assist clinical supervisors to remain current and competent?
- How feasible would it be to introduce these to your organisation?

Actively engaging in own supervision

It is essential that nurses who provide clinical supervision are actively involved in the process themselves. They should have their own clinical supervisor. The three main reasons for this are, firstly, engaging in clinical supervision ensures that supervisors have the professional support required to reflect on their roles, clinically and as a clinical supervisor. Secondly, one of the highest recommendations comes through one's own professional behaviours – clinical supervisors who have their own supervision role-model its importance. Supervisees may justifiably question the real value and importance of clinical supervision where the supervisor does not feel the need for it. Even experienced clinical supervisors will feel the strains and stresses associated with the role. Having their own clinical supervision is an important strategy for recognising and minimising supervisor burnout.

Finally, having clinical supervision yourself helps build your competency; you are in the position of inviting challenges, and questioning and reflecting on your own practice.

Recognising and overcoming supervisor burnout

The symptoms of burnout in clinical supervision are no different to the burnout experienced in other circumstances. People can experience both physical and emotional difficulties, which may or may not include headaches, sleep problems, gastrointestinal problems, chronic fatigue, grinding teeth, increased drug or alcohol use, muscle aches, high blood pressure, frequent colds, sudden weight loss or gain, apathy, frustration, difficulty concentrating, forgetfulness, depression, anger, negative or cynical attitude, being unexcited about life, inclination to high-risk behaviours, high emotional volatility and high irritability.

In the case of clinical supervisor, you may become alerted to the possibility of burnout when you begin to experience indifference towards one or more supervisees and their issues. The clinical supervisor experiencing burnout may find it difficult to get to sessions on time or look for easy excuses to cancel, particularly when working with certain supervisees. Within sessions burnout may manifest in supervisors having difficulty maintaining interest during the session, becoming irritated with the supervisee and feeling that nothing happening within the sessions makes the slight bit of difference.

It is crucial for supervisors to become aware of the symptoms and particularly the early warning signs so that support and assistance can be readily secured and appropriate strategies to overcome the problem or ensure a minimal impact can be implemented.

Potential causes of clinical supervisor burnout

There are certain factors that are likely to lead to clinical supervisor burnout.

- Supervisor not having their own clinical supervision and therefore not having adequate support for their supervisory role. Supervisors need the opportunity to reflect and explore their own role as clinical supervisors. Providing supervision is not always smooth sailing and supervisors are often confronted with ethical and legal issues or dilemmas. Having your own clinical supervisor is a necessary tool to support you.
- Clinical supervisors providing supervision for the organisation that employs them, but not having sufficient organisational support by way of policies and clear expectations for the role. Hence, supervisors can experience a heightened sense of vulnerability.
- Lack of adequate preparation for the role, resulting in the supervisor working outside the usual scope of practice, i.e. taking on responsibility for the supervisee's clinical practice where the supervisee should be accepting this responsibility.
- Difficulty maintaining clear boundaries around the supervisory session, which can lead to, for example, the supervisee requesting support and advice outside the structured session. Not being able to keep the supervision sessions boundaries clear and having trouble saying no when approaches are made outside the sessions.
- The experience of dual relationships. This is a particularly pertinent issue worthy of further discussion.

Dual relationships

A dual relationship, as the name suggests, means that the supervisor holds two roles in relation to the supervisee. Dual relationships present challenges for clinical supervision. This is not to suggest that all dual relationships are bad and should never occur, just that you need to always consider the potential for harm when there are dual relationships. Both the supervisor and the supervisee need to be aware of the duality. Prior to the commencement of supervision they should consider and discuss the issues that may arise and consider how they will manage the relationship when a conflict or difficulty arises.

There is at least one type of dual relationship that makes the supervisory relationship unworkable. This relates to line management. Management supervision and clinical supervision are two very different roles and should never be undertaken by the same person. With the combined manager/clinical supervisor role there is always an imbalance of power, the manager is responsible for the workplace the supervisee works in, including the staff, and this includes performance appraisal and performance management. If the manager is also the clinical supervisor this makes these conflicting roles impossible to manage.

Example

Janita is a highly experienced and well-respected nurse in the medical–surgical area. She has recently changed her career direction to the mental health field. Initially, she was completing a postgraduate course and received considerable assistance from preceptors and other clinical support staff in becoming skilled in this new field. Now that the course is completed she has indicated interest in receiving clinical supervision. Janita is assigned to David, the manager of the unit she is currently employed on. She has a fantastic relationship with David. He is enthusiastic, knowledgeable and encourages her to talk about her difficulties, but responds with encouragement and without any sense of disapproval. After a number of very positive sessions, Janita raises her concerns about a colleague of hers. Julie is an experienced mental health nurse who has worked with David for many years. Recently, Janita has become concerned at the relationship between the two of them. She feels that Julie likes to boss her around, does not provide clear direction and responds to Janita's questions by suggesting 'that's what books are for'.

Reflective exercise

- How would you feel to be David in this situation?
- What possible areas of conflict can you identify in this scenario?
- How would you approach the situation?

As a clinical supervisor it is David's role to explore the situation with Janita, encouraging her to consider her responses to Julie and how these behaviours or actions may possibly contribute to the conflict. He may suggest a number of communication strategies for future interactions. As a manager his imperatives will be quite different. David has serious concerns about Julie's level of ability and professionalism in her work. He is currently performance managing her. The testimony of Janita's experiences would probably strengthen his case that Julie should no longer be working in this area.

The two roles are in conflict: as a manager David wants to ensure he has the highest quality staff possible, which might encourage him to break confidentiality and report Janita's claim to his line manager in order to resolve a difficult staffing issue he has been working with. The desire to undertake this action is entirely understandable but it totally contravenes the purpose of clinical supervision. If he chose this course of action not only would David lose a potential opportunity to work with Janita to improve her skills in conflict management, he may well lose her trust and the trust of other colleagues. Janita may well feel her trust has been violated and may not feel comfortable receiving supervision from him any more. This creates an additional difficulty as she may fear that David will take a less positive view of her if she requests a change of supervisor.

The ramifications could become broader. It is quite likely that other nurses will become aware of the situation and develop (or increase) a negative attitude to clinical supervision.

There are a number of other dual relationships that have the potential for negative consequences but which are not so absolute as the line manager example. These additional relationships include:

- Close colleagues: Care needs to be taken if clinical supervision is to be provided where the supervisor and the colleague have worked closely together. The supervisor may find it difficult to maintain enough distance from the issues raised. For example, the supervisee is seeking advice and assistance in working with a long-term patient, commonly referred to as 'difficult' because of certain behavioural manifestations. The supervisor also knows the patient well and generally does not have a particularly positive view about her potential to achieve. At the very least this may mean the supervisor is less forthcoming with ideas and examples than would normally be the case. The outcome of issues may also have a direct impact on the clinical supervisor, therefore raising the potential for this to influence the clinical supervisor in his or her responses. Supervisors may inadvertently censor their responses in clinical supervision because of the potential impact for them.
- Friendship: The potential for conflict lies with both the friendship and the clinical supervision relationship. The clinical supervisor may find it difficult to challenge opinions, beliefs and actions if the supervisee is a friend. It may also be more difficult to maintain the level of formality required. As friends they may easily revert to 'chit chat' and lose the focus of their supervision. There is also a stronger possibility of griping about other colleagues, once again detracting from the purpose. If a clinical supervisory relationship does occur between friends, a clear agreement should be established with strict boundaries regarding the structure and content of sessions and a mutual agreement that the relationship be termi-

nated if either one or both of the parties feel it is no longer functioning effectively.

- Sexual relationships have similar issues to that of friendship, or possibly worse due to the tendency to consider that 'love is blind'. As we all know relationships do not always run smoothly, and any problems (temporary or longer term) will almost certainly influence the quality and effectiveness of clinical supervision. For example, if the couple are considering ending their relationship (particularly if this is the decision of one and not both), it would be difficult to put this issue aside and enter a clinical supervision session with an open and positive approach.

The imbalance of power and the potential for harm are quite high when clinical supervision enters the personal domain, making it difficult to maintain focus on the core activities of clinical supervision.

Reflective exercise

People often say that you should not mix friendship with business. However, even if we do not intentionally set out to work with friends, it is likely that we will develop friendships with colleagues at some stage in our professional careers. In many cases this causes little or no disruption to our working relationship. However, there may be occasions where you become concerned about your friend for some reason, such as coming to work late, not completing tasks on time, being abrasive at times or refusing to work with a specific nurse. You may be required to deal with this situation.

Consider an instance where this has happened to you and reflect on:

- how you felt about changing the role from one of friendship to one of authority
- how the way you felt in this situation differed to how you would feel in the same situation with a colleague with whom you did not have a close personal relationship
- how the friend/colleague responded to you
- the extent to which this response reflected your personal rather than professional relationship.

Consider the above situation in reverse, i.e. it is your friend that needed to speak with you about an aspect of your practice or performance and reflect on:

- how you felt with your friend being an authority figure in relation to your performance or practice
- the extent to which your reaction was influenced by your friendship.

If you found these situations difficult it is likely that the same issues will emerge in a clinical supervision setting. There are times you may need to challenge or possibly confront the supervisee and this can be difficult either because you find it difficult to relate to your friend other than in a friendly or cordial manner, or because your friend may become hurt or angry at such an approach and you do not want to risk a good friendship.

Your response may also vary from one friend to another. You may have friends who respond well to constructive criticism while others may not. The important thing is to consider the possible ramifications before you agree to providing clinical supervision where personal factors are involved. Remember you have the right to say no if someone asks you for clinical supervision and you do not believe it would be in the best interests of either or both of you to do this.

Role confusion: it is still your practice

Nurses and other health professionals may come to clinical supervision on the understanding that the supervisor is taking responsibility for clinical practice, that is the supervisee discusses the problem, the supervisor gives advice or instruction which the supervisee then carries out in practice, and if problems result the response may be 'that's what my clinical supervisor told me to do'. While clinical supervisors may be very clear about the scope and limitations of their role, supervisees may operate on the basis of very different assumptions. Clinical supervisors therefore need to be very clear that their role is not about decision-making or about taking responsibility for the clinical practice of the supervisees.

To avoid this pitfall, clinical supervisors need to have a sound understanding of the legal framework pertaining to the role (see Chapter 6). They also need to consider the impact of the context in which the clinical supervision occurs. There are important differences between providing clinical supervision within the organisation you work for and providing clinical supervision as part of your private practice. For example, people providing clinical supervision as an employee of an organisation will be expected to work in accordance with existing policies and procedures. It is quite likely that these policies and procedures were developed by people without an understanding of or experience in clinical supervision.

The clinical supervisor's familiarity with such policies and procedures is crucial in ensuring that the nurse works within the rules and regulations of the organisation. The clinical supervisor who works for the same organisation is likely to have a far greater knowledge in this respect than the clinical supervisor in private practice. If you are in private practice you may ask your supervisees for policies, mission statements, etc. to assist you to develop an understanding of the organisation they work in. Not only does this mean that as the clinical supervisor you are more likely to share similar knowledge of the organisational culture to the supervisee, but you may also then be in a more influential position to initiate or encourage changes to policies and procedures. You must always keep in mind where your knowledge came from as you do not want to compromise the integrity of the supervisory relationship.

Safety for clinical supervisors

Knowing yourself and owning your issues

Central to any effective clinical supervision process is investing time in developing self-awareness (clinical supervision for the supervisor is part of this). We can only be effective clinical supervisors when we are aware of what we also bring to the relationship. Self-understanding and knowledge help supervisors to maintain appropriate boundaries. For example, you may find it difficult to work effectively with a supervisee's distress when he or she is unable to make a decision or choose an appropriate course of action. By acknowledging and maintaining awareness of this you will be more likely when faced with a distressed supervisee to monitor your response rather than simply reverting to a natural tendency to provide reassurance and therefore deny the person the space and time to work through this distress.

Of course the same applies to you. Strong responses or reactions that you experience as a clinical supervisor should not be ignored but rather explored in your own clinical supervision. Some strong responses explored could provide you with a valuable insight into what is happening for the supervisee, for example as an indicator of transference (refer to Chapter 5). It may be useful to explore these with the supervisee or keep them to yourself for something that you observe and possibly monitor about yourself.

Often when we undertake new roles such as that of clinical supervisor, particularly if we have had little training or preparation, we tend to learn lessons the hard way, that is we do not truly appreciate the situations we are likely to find difficult until we encounter them. Given the example above, the fact that we tend to want to comfort and reassure people in distress is not likely to surprise us. It is sure to feature strongly in our personal relationships and professional encounters with both staff and patients. However, it is quite possible that we will not even consider this in relation to clinical supervision until it happens.

This is not the end of the world and there is much capacity to learn from and through clinical supervision but it may be useful to anticipate personality characteristics that you feel may present a barrier to your role as a clinical supervisor.

Reflective exercise

Consider some of your traits or characteristics that may be unhelpful in various aspects of your life on both a personal and a professional basis. Consider how these traits may limit the effectiveness of your clinical supervision skills and, finally, think about some of the ways you might contain them. This would be useful to explore with your own clinical supervisor before you commence this role yourself.

Dealing with problems in the supervisory relationship

In the role of clinical supervisor you are on one level expected to be able to address conflict and have the capacity to discuss issues that you believe need to be discussed. You are the one who is facilitating a process that enables supervisees to see things they may not have otherwise seen. As we know, you are also human and have your own issues and ways of dealing with conflict. It is important that you have an understanding of how you manage conflict generally.

Reflective exercise

Consider and reflect on the following questions:

- What are the things that get in the way of you addressing difficult issues with people you know?
- Are you able to let people know if you are disappointed or hurt, etc.?
- How do you address these issues? Do you consider the way you manage things to be helpful or destructive?
- How do you think those closest to you would answer the above questions?

Being a clinical supervisor is a complex and rewarding role. It is not a passive role. You need to ensure that you are both adequately prepared and supported, in order that you can maximise your value for the supervisees. Understanding yourself and dealing with your own issues is an important part of this process.

The clinical supervisee

Choosing the right supervisor for you

In Chapter 3 we considered the implementation of clinical supervision in a mental health service in rural Victoria. One of the strategies used was to develop a folder with information about each of the clinical supervisors. The aim was to enable supervisees to make an informed choice about the supervisor they would prefer. This strategy was highly successful, and had the additional benefit of increasing the profile of clinical supervision. A folder is a tangible item; it has a physical presence and may therefore be more influential in spreading the word about clinical supervision than verbal communication.

The concept of informed choice is an important one for nursing and health care; we respect the importance of patients receiving frank and honest information about their physical or psychological status and having the opportunity to make autonomous decisions from the range of treatment options available. Informed choice is no less important in clinical supervision. The information folder described in Chapter 3 recognises the importance of informed choice and of the importance of the relationship in clinical supervision.

Since clinical supervision has been introduced into nursing relatively recently, it is not likely that most health care services will have developed an information folder. Nevertheless, it is important that you find the right clinical supervisor for you. Sometimes nurses assume that because a nurse is an excellent clinician or educator he or she will also make an excellent clinical supervisor. This is not necessarily the case and even nurses we might class as excellent supervisors will not suit everybody. That is why it is important that you make your own informed decision.

Reflective exercise

Consider the information you would like about potential supervisors. If you are receiving supervision or have done so previously you can probably answer this from your own personal experience.

The following list presents information supervisees commonly find useful to know about supervisors:

- discipline (e.g. nursing, allied health)
- specialisation, e.g. medical or surgical, emergency, midwifery, mental health
- current role
- nursing background:
  ○ years of experience
  ○ additional qualifications
  ○ specific skills and interests, for example psychodrama
- experience as a clinical supervisor
- clinical supervision style, for example active experiential approach, likes using role-plays
- knowledge and skill in specific clinical supervision models, e.g. solution focused, psychodynamic.

Reflective exercise

Supervisor wanted.

*   Write one to two paragraphs describing the characteristics you would want in a clinical supervisor.
*   Separate out the desirable from the essential (if possible – they may all be essential).

If you have colleagues who have previously engaged in clinical supervision show them your advertisement and ask:

*   Is there anything they think you have missed?
*   How likely is it that you would be able to find someone with all or most of those characteristics?

Do not throw this exercise away. It might provide a useful basis on which to conduct an interview with potential supervisors in the future.

It is important that you do not feel pressured to select a supervisor because others tell you he or she is great or because you are worried you might hurt a person's feelings if you choose someone else. This is an important relationship and it must work for you. First and foremost you need to know that your clinical supervisor has his or her own clinical supervisor. It is also useful to know how long he or she has been having clinical supervision and whether his or her understanding of the process is the result of being a participant in supervision. Receiving supervision provides a very important learning environment for people wanting to become supervisors. However, experience of this type is influenced by the quality of the supervisor. This is particularly pertinent when your supervisor has only received supervision from the one person. In this situation there is a tendency to model one's own approach on individual experience, without the advantage of being able to compare this approach to others.

You may also want to know how long the supervisor has been providing supervision. However, it should not be simply a matter of deciding that more experience equates to better skills. Everybody has to start somewhere. You may find that a person providing clinical supervision for the first time is an excellent supervisor. He or she may have the capacity to draw on experience in the clinical area and from being a supervisee. It is important to consider the person's broader skill range because a number of factors influence the capacity to be an effective clinical supervisor. It is important that prospective supervisors can discuss their qualifications and experience for the role frankly. It is crucial that you both have a sense of each other's skill base and experience.

Choosing a clinical supervisor is personal. Some people look for someone who is similar in style to themselves, others look for someone with contrasting skills. People do, however, generally seek someone they respect personally and professionally. Your clinical supervisor needs to be someone with whom you could share sensitive material, someone you could tolerate feeling vulnerable with and trust that you would be treated with respect at all times. Despite the person's style you will need to have a supervisor who is prepared to challenge you and has the capacity to help you explore a range of possibilities in a supportive setting rather than simply accepting your perspective.

Dealing with problems in the supervisory relationship from the perspective of the supervisee

It can be difficult to raise any concerns or problems you are having with clinical supervision. For this reason it is especially important to discuss processes for managing difficulties at the commencement of the supervisory relationship. In this early stage the relationship should be free of difficulties, therefore providing an opportunity to discuss ways to deal with conflict when it is an abstract concept rather than a reality.

Once the relationship has been established there are a number of issues that can prevent problems being addressed, including:

- not wanting to upset or offend the supervisor – a particular problem for supervisees who like their supervisor
- fear or apprehension that the supervisor will respond in a way that could threaten the supervisory relationship
- lack of confidence in own judgement that makes the supervisee reluctant to question the supervisor.

As discussed earlier in this chapter, in relation to supervisors, it is helpful to reflect on the way you deal with conflict in other aspects of your life. You will more than likely deal with issues in clinical supervision in a similar way. The following exercise can assist you in identifying your approach to conflict.

Reflective exercise

- If a friend does something that really bothers you how do you manage it? Are you able to talk about how you feel?
- If conditions at work change and impact on you negatively, what would you do? Would you tolerate the situation or would you be able to let people know of the impact? Would you simply resign without giving a reason?
- When you reveal your feelings do you become angry and raise your voice? Or are you calm and able to speak your mind but also listen to the other person?

This is by no means a complete list, but rather a guide to assist you in thinking about how you deal with conflict. Ideally, this should be discussed with your supervisor. If you are able to discuss how you are likely to manage any conflict, then together you can work out how to manage it. This may also leave you feeling that you have been given permission to discuss issues as they arise.

Making the most of clinical supervision

Throughout this book considerable attention has been devoted to describing the value and uses of clinical supervision. Previous chapters provide an overview of approaches to clinical supervision such as group or individual, and give consideration to issues such as whether or not clinical supervision should be discipline specific (see Chapter 4). Those readers who have previously experienced clinical supervision will hopefully already have positive opinions about the impact of clinical supervision on practice. However, not all nurses have had clinical supervision, some have never heard of the term or confuse it with others such as preceptorship and performance management (see Chapter 1). For nurses who have had clinical supervision not all experiences have been positive. Nurses come to supervision for a variety of reasons and it is not always voluntary. Before you can fully consider what you might achieve from clinical supervision, it is important to reflect on what has brought you to this point.

Reflective exercise

Take the time to consider and answer the following questions:

- Who made the decision for you to start clinical supervision?
  - If it was your decision:
    - What factors motivated or influenced you?
    - Why do you want clinical supervision?
  - If it was not your decision how do you feel about being coerced or persuaded into it?
- Have you had clinical supervision before? If so, what was your previous experience like?
- Do you already have some idea about what you are hoping to get out of clinical supervision? What are your expectations?

In asking and answering these questions you may begin to develop an understanding about what you bring to the relationship and whether the impact is likely to be positive or negative. If you feel that you were pressured or coerced into having clinical supervision then the clinical supervisor is likely to be working with the negative feelings that you have, such as anger, anxiety or mistrust. On the other hand, if you chose to engage in clinical supervision because you believe it will provide an opportunity to reflect on and work towards developing your practice, your supervisor is likely to be working with a high level of enthusiasm and motivation.

You will also bring with you any previous experience of clinical supervision. For example, if you have had supervision previously with a very directive supervisor who tended to provide solutions about how to manage situations you presented, you may well come to supervision with a similar expectation of your new supervisor, tending to wait for the same level of direction. If the new supervisor's style is not directive you may come to experience this as withholding information. This is a form of projection called transference (see Chapter 5). The supervisee projects his or her expectations onto the supervisor and becomes confused when the supervisor does not respond according to expectations. Having a level of self-awareness can assist you to develop a clearer relationship with your supervisor, it will not necessarily stop you having those expectations but you may recognise where they come from and allow you to discuss them openly with your supervisor.

Education and training

Earlier in this chapter the importance of education and training was discussed in relation to clinical supervisors. The need for educational preparation for supervisors has been addressed in the literature (McKeown, 2001; Clifton, 2002; Hancox et al., 2004). However, no similar attention has been paid to the educational preparation for supervisees. Clinical supervision is widely regarded as being associated with a number of myths and misconceptions and nurses have been found to view this process as 'snoopervision' (Yegdich, 1999), and therefore often view the process with suspicion and concern.

As stated previously the role of supervisee should not be seen as a passive one. If supervisees are active participants in the supervisory relationship then surely education is as important for supervisees as it is for supervisors. Education could potentially assist to inform supervisees about the nature of clinical supervision and the benefits they can expect from it. It provides an opportunity to dispel common myths and misconceptions, and to equip supervisees with the skills and knowledge they require to be active participants in the supervision relationship.

Nursing specific vs multidisciplinary supervision

There is often debate about whether nurses should receive supervision from other nurses, or whether it is reasonable and justifiable to seek supervision from another member of the multidisciplinary team. However, this debate is probably less productive than is considering what one hopes to gain from clinical supervision. Being clear about your goals should guide you in the selection of the most appropriate supervisor. For example, if you hope to improve your skills and knowledge about family therapy, there would be little point in seeking supervision from a nurse with little knowledge or experience in family therapy in preference to a social worker with considerable expertise in this area. Your choice of supervisor would probably be more appropriately addressed by considering what you hope to achieve rather than following a set of predetermined rules.

Conclusion

The relationship between supervisor and supervisee is central to the success of clinical supervision. In order to maximise the positive impact of this relationship, it is crucial that both supervisors and supervisees are well prepared for their respective roles. This chapter has provided a detailed examination of the roles of clinical supervisor and supervisee, including the skills and knowledge required for effective supervision. Given the importance of this relationship it is important to ensure a good match between the two parties to the relationship and that strategies are put in place to deal with potential conflicts in the supervisory relationship.

References

Bond, M. & Holland, S. (1998) *Skills of Supervision for Nurses*. Oxford: Open University Press.

Clifton, E. (2002) Implementing clinical supervision. *Nursing Times*, 98(9), 36–37.

Department of Health, Western Australia (2005) *Clinical Supervision: Framework for WA Mental Health Services and Clinicians*. Perth: Department of Health, Western Australia.

Department of Human Services, Victoria (2006) Guidelines for clinical supervision. Retrieved August 2006 from www.dhs.vic.gov.au/mentalhealth.

Hancox, K., Lynch, L., Happell, B. & Biondo, S. (2004) An evaluation of an educational program for clinical supervision. *International Journal of Mental Health Nursing*, 13(3), 198–203.

McKeown, C. (2001) Find time for supervision. *Nursing Standard*, 16(2), 25–27.

Yegdich, T. (1999) Clinical supervision and managerial supervision: Some historical and conceptual considerations. *Journal of Advanced Nursing*, 30(5), 1195–1204.

Clinical supervision in action

Introduction

Clinical supervision is about much more than a couple of people in a room chatting. It is an important relationship that must be taken seriously if it is to fulfil its promise. The aim of this chapter is to provide guidance in preparing for the establishment of a supervisory relationship, including:

- the Hancox/Lynch model of clinical supervision
- the development of clinical supervision agreements
- how to conduct the first session
- conducting subsequent clinical supervision sessions.

The Hancox/Lynch model of clinical supervision

Throughout this text we have been discussing the many and complex factors that comprise and influence clinical supervision. We have considered what clinical supervision is and what it is not, provided a model to guide the implementation process, explored the various approaches available, and considered some of the models that can guide the clinical supervision relationship. Legal issues and ethical issues have been considered and the important roles of the supervisor and supervisee have been examined in detail. It is likely you now feel you know a lot more about clinical supervision. However, how to actually do clinical supervision may still be a mystery to many of you. Despite reading this text some of you may still be wondering what you do once you have decided to take on the role of a clinical supervisor.

In this chapter, the Hancox/Lynch model of clinical supervision will be presented. This model provides a structure for conducting clinical supervision sessions and demonstrates the benefits of following a framework for clinical supervision. This model assists beginning supervisors to establish a sound structure to support their practice as supervisors. The model was developed by Hancox and Lynch as the result of over a decade of experience as providers and teachers of clinical supervision. Through their experiences the authors recognised a gap between understanding the theory and applying the practice of clinical supervision. Gaining more detailed information about the models of clinical supervision helped to explore the purpose and desired outcomes of clinical supervision but did not necessarily demonstrate the 'how to' or 'clinical supervision in action'. The following section will provide a comprehensive overview of the Hancox/Lynch model and walk you step by step through the process of supervision, from the point at which you commit to becoming a clinical supervisor.

The information and reflective exercises in Chapter 7 should have assisted your preparation as a clinical supervisor. Hopefully you now have an understanding of why you want to be a clinical supervisor and what motivates you to take on this responsible role.

Reflective exercise

Refer back to the advert you wrote to describe yourself:

- Why might someone choose you as a clinical supervisor?
- What skills, knowledge and experience do you offer?

Ask four colleagues you trust and respect to read the advert and tell you honestly (on the basis of the advert rather than what they already know about you):

- if they would choose you as a clinical supervisor
- if so, what particular aspects of your description would make them consider you as a suitable supervisor
- if not, what aspects of the description would deter them from selecting you
- what, if any, important information you have left out of the description.

As mentioned above, you may be committed to becoming a clinical supervisor, you may have completed a training program and have increased your knowledge at a theoretical level, but how do you actually do it? The Hancox/Lynch model has two interacting parts: knowledge and relationship. These essential parts are encompassed within a context. The context is the overlay that contextualises and influences all elements of clinical supervision and its importance cannot be underestimated. The model is represented below as an infinity symbol (refer to Figure 8.1). The use of the infinity symbol is intended to represent

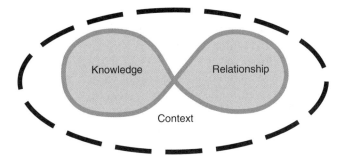

Figure 8.1 The Hancox/Lynch model of clinical supervision in action.

the potentially ongoing nature of clinical supervision, the fact that it has no predefined end date. Unlike preceptorship, which has a pre-assigned time frame, clinical supervision is constantly evaluated, constantly reviewed and continues until either the supervisor or the supervisee ends it. For this reason the sign of the infinity was seen as the most accurate pictorial representation.

The main elements of the model are encircled with the context. Here the context surrounds the infinity sign with a dotted line that forms a circle. Again this is symbolic: the circle does not have a clearly defined beginning and end, it is ongoing and never ending. This again reminds us that the context is always important and should always be considered within the supervisory relationship. The dotted line is similar to that of a semipermeable membrane as it allows constant movement. Context is not static; it is a dynamic phenomenon that is formed by ever-changing influences. Thinking about the supervisory relationship within the context of the supervisee's world will be a concept familiar to most nurses. Nurses are trained to consider the whole person within the system in which they live.

Example

Jeff is a 23-year-old man brought to the emergency department following a serious motor vehicle accident. No major organ or bone damage has been detected but Jeff has sustained burns and abrasions to his face, neck and arms. As a nurse in this setting you would recognise the importance of treating the physical injuries, providing pain relief and avoiding the risk of infection. However, you would also recognise the importance of psychosocial support. Jeff can see the burns and other injuries to his arms, he can feel the pain from his face and neck and is concerned that he will be physically disfigured for life. He refuses to see his girlfriend, who was driving the car at the time of the accident, and is visibly distressed by what she 'has done to him'. Promoting recovery for Jeff means doing the very best to meet all of his needs.

The same is true for clinical supervision. It is not possible to sit in a room with a supervisee and black out every part of that person other than that which directly relates to nursing practice. The supervisee will be influenced by many factors that shape his or her experiences and attitudes – religious and ethical values, ability to relate to patients and colleagues, and confidence in dealing with particular situations will all be influenced by educational preparation, length and diversity of experience, and a host of personality factors.

Interestingly, as nurses we are often far more understanding of the patient as part of a total system than we are of our nursing colleagues. While we make allowances for less than desirable behaviour or actions from patients who have suffered a traumatic event, we may regard a nurse in the same situation as unprofessional or not having 'what it takes' to be a nurse. In conducting clinical supervision sessions it is important that supervisors allow their supervisees to expose their 'humanness', to feel sufficiently confident that they will not be judged to disclose insecurities and issues of concern. It is important to remember that clinical supervision is not therapy (see Chapter 1), yet understand the complexity of nurses as people and appreciate how personal factors can influence professional practice.

Nursing also requires a systemic approach to the delivery of care; nurses are required to juggle the competing needs of colleagues, patients and families, and navigate management and bureaucratic processes to ensure the best outcomes for their patients. Considering the context is essential!

Context

The context surrounding clinical supervision is of outmost importance, and as highlighted above it is dynamic and ever-changing. Whilst it is all-encompassing, for the sake of further examination, the context of clinical supervision can be broken into three main parts: the beginning, the role, and the organisation or system in which the nurse works.

The beginning refers specifically to the establishment of the supervisory relationship – the first contacts, the first sessions, those early encounters that are focused on establishing rapport and a firm foundation. The second part refers to the role of the supervisee, who he or she is, what position he or she holds, his or her role and why is it important for this to be known within clinical supervision. The third part refers to the organisation. More specifically it is concerned with the exploration and understanding of the world in which the supervisee works. While it is important to define the concepts of role and organisation in the beginning this will constantly change, constantly be affected by change and constantly structure or frame the context around your supervisee and the clinical supervision sessions. It does not matter whether you are providing clinical supervision as an internal or an external clinical supervisor, it is important to develop an understanding of the organisation in which the supervisees are working.

We will explore each of the subsections on context below in detail; however, to assist you as a new supervisor we will start with the exploration of context around beginning the clinical supervision relationship.

The beginning

So what is the context that surrounds the establishment of the clinical supervisory relationship and how can focusing on the context assist you in setting up supervision? The context surrounding the beginning of clinical supervision is focused on what brings the supervisee to supervision. This can be explored in the following ways.

The context surrounding the first contact for supervision
The first contact for clinical supervision is about both parties getting to know each other and beginning to form the relationship. The way this beginning phase transpires will depend on whether this is the first time you have met or whether you had a prior relationship. When supervision is provided by a member of staff from the same organisation, it is possible you have previously worked in a collegial fashion. The context becomes one of obverting previous relationships and exploring the possible implications. If you have never met previously, your only former contact may have been by phone or email. In this situation, the context becomes one of establishing a relationship and mutual understanding.

The context surrounding the first supervision session
While there are some important tasks to complete in the first session, the main focus is the formation of the relationship. As the supervisor your role is to engage with the supervisee and begin to establish rapport, whilst at the same time setting the boundaries and parameters. This can often take considerable time and should not be rushed. For this reason we recommend between 1 and 1½ hours for the first session.

Think back to Chapter 7, where the roles of the supervisor and supervisee were articulated. Some of the information we discussed in those chapters forms the basis for the tasks you will need to complete in this first session. Again think back to your advertisement, what the supervisee needs or wants to know about you. You may even feel comfortable asking supervisees why they chose you for supervision. There are also a number of things you identified in the previous chapters that you wanted to know about supervisees: their characteristics, such as discipline and professional background, education and training, including any education in clinical supervision, and their strengths and struggles as clinicians. This is also the time to explore past experiences with supervision. Has their experience been positive or negative, and what, if any, influence or even leftover baggage does this bring to this supervision experience? Depending on their experiences with supervision this exploration may take a bit of time. That is okay, you are establishing the structures of the relationship and it is important to spend time ensuring that these initial structures have firm foundations.

The first session may begin by asking the supervisee to provide an overview of his or her:

- role within the organisation, both professional and otherwise, for example the supervisee may also be the union representative
- reasons for selecting you as supervisor
- previous experience with supervision and how he or she is currently influenced by those experiences.

Where the supervisee's previous experiences have been negative, hard work is needed to establish the type of relationship that will facilitate the supervisee to actively become involved in the process, recognise it is not the same as previous experiences and begin to see the process more positively.

Example

Sonya commences a clinical supervision session with Robert. She has not worked with Robert before, and during their first session she finds that Robert is a Grade 2 nurse with about 5 years' experience in nursing. Two years ago he was involved in group clinical supervision in the unit he worked on. At that time Robert was not very popular with his colleagues. He was the newest to the team and there was a general sense from others that he had no respect for existing processes. During supervision sessions Robert was often the source of criticism. From Roberts's perspective this conflict was not well addressed by the group clinical supervisor. Consequently, Robert terminated his involvement in clinical supervision and left the organisation. He took with him a very negative and resentful attitude to clinical supervision. He has been pressured to be involved in this instance and is not expecting positive outcomes.

Sonya's first reaction may be, 'Oh no, what can I do here to overcome these negative attitudes?' The first thing is to acknowledge Robert's previous experience. Take care to avoid statements like 'I don't think that could be right, clinical supervision isn't like this'. This is not to suggest you need to agree with everything Robert has said. The important thing is to ask Robert about the situation from his perspective, and how he felt it could have been dealt with more effectively to enable him to feel more comfortable and protected within the process. This alone is likely to increase Robert's confidence that this clinical supervisor is respectful and supportive. Furthermore, Sonya could ask Robert what he needs to feel safe and comfortable in his current clinical supervision. This could form the beginning of a relationship based on trust and mutual respect.

The context in which the clinical supervision has begun
It is essential to understand the motivation of the supervisee. For example, the supervisee might state the following: 'I want clinical supervision because I am going for a new position and my manager thought it would be helpful for me to explore my practice' or 'I have experienced clinical supervision in my previous employment and have found it really beneficial. I wanted the opportunity to experience it again.' In these two examples the supervisee describes different motivations for seeking supervision: one example is influenced by an external motivator, namely to respond to the wishes of the manager, the other is an internal motivation, based on the supervisee's experience of clinical supervision as a helpful process.

It may be easy to conclude that internal motivators are preferable to the external; however, in reality both external and internal motivators could be malignant or benign. There may be negative or malignant forces that influence someone to seek out clinical supervision. For example, managers may pressure their staff to access supervision because of performance issues (external) or a supervisee may engage in clinical supervision for something to add to their CV to improve the likelihood of promotion, rather than because of perceived benefits (internal). On the other hand managers may actively work towards creating a culture where nurses are able to access clinical supervision. They may encourage staff to attend and perhaps even offer inducements (such as free movie tickets) for nurses to give it a try, reflecting the view that nurses may need an external motivation to start the process, but that ultimately they will recognise the benefits and attend because they consider the experience to be intrinsically valuable. As a clinical supervisor it is important to explore this motivation in detail to provide you with a comprehensive understanding of the context in which clinical supervision has commenced.

What do the expectations of supervisees bring to the context of
the clinical supervision?
A further advantage of exploring the motivation of supervisees is that it provides further insight into their expectations. It is important to spend some time in order to really understand what it is the supervisee is wanting from the supervision. This level of understanding enables the supervisee and supervisor to discuss the extent to which the expectations are realistic and reasonable.

In some situations supervisees may not be clear about their motivation for seeking supervision and may be even less clear about their expectations. Achieving this level of clarity takes time. Supervisees should be encouraged to reflect on their motivations and expectations. It is also important that this not be seen as a preliminary step. Clinical supervision is a long-term process and therefore it is neither important nor possible to identify all the expectations the supervisee has and compile a detailed list of goals and expectations in the first session. It is just the beginning. However, a comprehensive understanding of the expectations is crucial to the success of a supervisory relationship. If the time spent in supervision does not have any obvious aims, purpose or outcomes, nurses will be likely to resist or withdraw from active involvement in the process.

Clinical supervisors need to identify their roles as facilitative rather than directive. It is crucial that supervisees explore their own expectations, set their own goals and take responsibility for them. In some instances supervisees may encourage or even try to push the supervisor to take an active role in defining their supervision goals. Such a passive approach is to be avoided. The primary aim of clinical supervision is to enhance the professional and clinical development of individual nurses. It must therefore be directed by supervisees towards the outcomes and skill development that are valuable for them. They need to drive clinical supervision and set their own agendas, not merely follow what has been set by the clinical supervisor.

The activity below provides a framework for you as the supervisor to assist supervisees in identifying the goals they hope to achieve from clinical supervision.

Reflective exercise

- Which specialties of nursing interest you most?
- What draws you to these specialties?
- Where do you see yourself professionally in 5 years' time?
- What do you need to do to achieve these professional goals?
- What have been some of the past barriers and supports to you in achieving your professional goals?
- What do you think would be your future barriers and supports?
- How do you see clinical supervision supporting this?

Once you are clearer about what has brought the supervisee to supervision, and what he or she wants to get out of it, you can then move towards formulating the clinical supervision agreement.

The clinical supervision agreement

So what is a clinical supervision agreement? Like all relationships, clinical supervision requires boundaries to ensure it achieves its aims and does not become sidetracked into a different type of relationship. The clinical supervision agreement is one safeguard. The agreement provides a written account of mutually understood expectations of the process, endorsed by both parties. It provides a context for the clinical supervision by providing the foundations, framework and overall structure. In a very basic way the agreement provides a useful checklist that assists the supervisor and supervisee to clarify and cement the boundaries of the relationship and ensure all necessary information is discussed and understood, so that a common understanding of the supervision is gained. You both know what you are agreeing to (Beinart, 2004).

The supervision agreement helps to prepare the supervisor and supervisee for clinical supervision. It is formed by both parties and provides a map for the entire supervisory experience. Clinical supervision agreements are a practical and essential supervision tool. They highlight the commitment of both supervisors and supervisees to the clinical supervision process. However, supervisees may not immediately see this. Nurses often react with fear or suspicion when it is time to form and sign the actual agreement. This is quite understandable. Think of the last time you signed your name to a document. Many people dislike or feel suspicious about signing documents. Often this can make us feel compelled or coerced, like we are binding ourselves to some type of legal contract. Most of the documents we sign in our lifetime signify long-term commitments and legal obligations. Marriage certificates, contract of sale, loan papers or leases are documents we do not take lightly because of the generally long-term nature of the commitment involved and potentially serious consequences if we are not able to fulfil the requirements. The requirement to sign an agreement may suddenly change supervisees' attitudes by propelling clinical supervision to a more formal, possibly even legally binding, relationship. These feelings can actually be intensified when the supervision is occurring within the workplace; supervision agreements can feel like a form of management surveillance, more akin to the 'snoopervision' that fuelled many of the myths and misconceptions about supervision that were explored in Chapter 1.

In the role of clinical supervisor you are likely to understand the purpose and intention of clinical supervision agreements. However, it is important not to dismiss the concerns of supervisees. Be prepared to spend time discussing the agreement and its purpose. Do not pressure supervisees to sign, they must feel comfortable to do so. Encourage questions and answer them honestly and thoughtfully.

What is included in a supervision agreement?
Supervisors should design a template for supervision agreements containing all of the essentials with parts of the agreement left blank to be completed in consultation with the supervisee. The agreement needs to include many of the fundamentals we have explored throughout this text. The suggestions below are intended to assist supervisors to develop agreements; they are not exhaustive and should not be taken as a universal template. It is important for supervisors to design their own agreements, but hopefully the following suggested components of clinical supervision will be helpful:

- A definition of clinical supervision or a description of its overall aim, purpose or function. This will assist in clarifying what clinical supervision is, what the purpose of the relationship is and what the supervisee hopes to achieve. It could even be a summary statement of your explorations together during the first part of the first session when you were getting to know each other and clarifying motivations and expectations. Refer back to Chapter 6, particularly to the issue of informed consent. For someone to be able to give informed consent they must understand what it is they are consenting to. A clear definition that articulates what you as a supervisor mean for clinical supervision can assist you to do this.
- Issues not appropriate to discuss in clinical supervision. This is about clarifying the boundaries of what is and is not appropriate to focus on in supervision. This will be a broad statement rather than specific detail. However, it needs to include a statement keeping the focus on the professional context, for example *'Clinical supervision is about exploring your professional life, the focus is on you, within the context of your role at work as a nurse. It is not a forum for you to discuss or explore personal issues that have no influence or impact on your work life. Sometimes the line between work and home is not as clear cut as we would like, as there are many instances when personal issues affect your role at work. Together we will tease out these situations and openly discuss whether this is work related or more personal. As your supervisor I can assist you to seek personal support via counselling if you would like.'*
- Expectations of clinical supervisor and supervisee. This is likely to include statements such as:
  - the supervision sessions are directed by supervisees and focused on their particular needs
  - the supervisee must be prepared and ready to make the most of each session
  - supervisees may be required to undertake specific tasks between sessions, for example practice assertive skills with their line manager
- Make specific reference to the professional code of ethics or standards for practice. Explicitly acknowledge the Code of Ethics and Professional Standards that regulate nursing practice to assist in focusing on the potential ethical and legal issues that may arise
- Reviewing and concluding the supervisory relationship. The process for reviewing the supervisory relationship and how one or both parties can conclude clinical supervision when necessary needs to be clearly articulated in the agreement. Review should be a regular part of the supervisory relationship and the time period for review should be agreed to by both parties. Reviews may occur after every 10 sessions or 3 monthly or 6 monthly. The review provides an opportunity for both parties to consider the strength of the

relationship and the extent to which the supervisee's goals are being realised. Do not leave reviewing the relationship to only when and if things are not 'travelling well'. Ensure there are planned review processes and ensure that these are strictly adhered to.

- Specific policies and procedures relating to clinical supervision that are present within the organisation. Often these organisational policies will focus on the legal and ethical issues and may include:
  - confidentiality and its legal limitations
  - storage of notes
  - conflict resolution process
  - mandatory reporting
  - staff/patient boundaries.

It is not possible in an agreement to explain all of the above policies in detail. By referring to them or attaching them to the agreement the supervisor can ensure that the supervisee is aware that the policies exist and can refer to them as required.

The following is an example of a clinical supervision agreement based on one formulated by clinical supervision consultants. This agreement applies to provision from within an organisation. An additional suggestion for appropriate agreements if the supervision is offered privately is also included.

Example of a clinical supervision agreement

'Clinical supervision is a formal process of consultation between two or more professionals. The focus is to provide support for the supervisee(s) in order to promote self-awareness, development and growth within the context of their professional environment.' (Hancox & Lynch, 2002)

I (name of supervisee) _____ will attend clinical supervision sessions with (name of supervisor) _____ commencing on (date of first session) _____ these sessions will be weekly/fortnightly/monthly (strike out inapplicable).

They will be 1-hour duration at a time and place negotiated and suiting both parties. Where possible confidentiality will be assured by both parties, however should information of a confidential nature need to be disclosed for clinical or legal reasons, both parties will be given the opportunity to discuss the terms of the disclosure. Where possible the clinical supervisor will act as a support person or advocate for the supervisee.

The clinical supervisor will keep process notes on all sessions; the nature of these notes and storage of them is outlined below and agreed on by both parties.

_____

_____

Continued

Note: Your organisation has stated that they do not want access to the supervision notes and have agreed that they are the private property of the supervisor and the supervisee. Although unlikely, legally notes maybe required in court or by the Nurses' Board in the case of an investigation into conduct.

Reviewing the clinical supervision session should occur at the times agreed on below. However, either party can raise difficulties or issues pertaining to supervision at anytime.

_____
_____

Whilst I understand that emergencies in the workplace occur and we need to be flexible, the supervisee agrees to give as much notice as possible if a session is to be cancelled. The contact number is: _____

Together we have discussed and reviewed your Professional Code of Conduct for your profession and the relevant policies and procedures related to clinical supervision are as follows:

Clinical supervision for nurses
Confidentiality and its legal limitations, including mandatory reporting
Ownership and storage of clinical supervision notes
Conflict resolution process
Staff/client boundaries

These policies are available on the intranet and in the policy and procedure manual in your workplace. Please ensure that you have read and are familiar with these policies and procedures. If you have any concerns please do not hesitate to raise them with me and we can note any issues below.

_____
_____

The supervisee's expectations and overall goals of clinical supervision are:

_____
_____
_____

Any further points of discussion

_____
_____
_____
_____

Signed and dated
Supervisor _____   Supervisee _____

If you are conducting supervision privately your clinical supervision agreement may be quite a bit shorter than the organisational one above. Whilst many of the overall concepts still apply, there are some main differences:

(1) Notes are owned by the supervisor.
(2) The supervisee agrees to give 24 hours' notice if a session is to be cancelled. If this does not occur, fees will still apply.
(3) There are no organisational policies or procedures, so individual agreement on these issues needs to be negotiated privately.

Both parties should hold a copy of this agreement. In some organisations it is an expectation that all clinical supervision agreements are stored in a specific location. The organisation may choose to use clinical supervision agreements as a way to demonstrate their commitment to clinical support of their staff. For example, they may need to demonstrate for accreditation that they provide clinical supervision or it may be specified that all clinical supervision arrangements supported by this particular organisation must have an agreement, thereby ensuring that the organisation's, supervisors' and supervisees' understanding of what is meant by clinical supervision is similar.

Reflective exercise

Are there any other factors that have not been mentioned that you feel should be included in a supervision agreement in your workplace? What are they and why are they important?

List all the things you want to include in your own personal clinical supervision agreement.

Now write your own clinical supervision agreement. How similar or different is your agreement from the examples provided in this text?

This exploration during the first sessions and the development and signing of the clinical supervision agreement defines the context of the initial clinical supervision relationship. Whilst context continues to provide the essential overlay throughout every session, the initial foundation has now been laid. This ground work provides the basis to explore the broader context of role and organisation. This can be started almost immediately after the initial 'getting to know you' sessions, and following the writing and signing of the clinical supervision agreement.

Role

The role refers to the professional position the supervisee holds and the roles and responsibilities that accompany it. The concept of role is complex and organisationally shaped. It is also individually shaped. The individual brings his or her personality, which in turn influences the individual interpretation of the role and its functions. There can be discord between an individual's interpretation of a role and the vision of the organisation. A role exists within an organisation and an individual exists beyond an organisation. It is the role that creates the connection between the individual and the organisation. Without the role the individual's place in the organisation is not defined (Borwick, 2006). As a clinical supervisor it is therefore very important to develop an understanding of the roles the supervisees hold and how they view them. What is the nature of their connection to the organisation?

Important considerations for the context of role:

- Refer to the job description for the role at its inception. This can be an interesting exercise, especially if someone has been in a workplace and role for a long time. The role often develops and moves a little away from what it was initially. Looking at what it was and exploring what it has been can help the supervisee become aware of how this has changed, why it has changed, what the influences were that led to the change and whether the changes now best suit their environment.
- A stocktake of roles and portfolios in addition to the supervisee's designated role. This involves the identification of further roles and functions and whether these have developed from individual interest or by a request from management. For example, a staff member may be employed in the role of associate nurse unit manager (ANUM) but has taken on the role of union representative out of interest. Using these two roles as an example, the clinical supervisor may want to know if whether holding these two roles is problematic. The manager of the ANUM may find the presence of the ANUM as a union representative positive because of his or her desire to consult closely with the union. On the other hand, the unit manager may feel threatened by this dual role and feel that the role of union representative prevents the supervisee from effectively executing his or her responsibilities as an ANUM.
- Which roles do supervisees intend to work on in clinical supervision?
- Boundaries of the role? How are these boundaries known? What authority does the supervisee have in the role? What is their understanding of their role?

There are a number of ways you may work with a supervisee to explore these issues. You might like to ask them to do a projective drawing like the one described in Chapter 5 under Systems psychodynamics, or you may take a curious position, asking them questions and assisting them to reflect on their role as they answer you.

Example

Supervisor: You say you are the ANUM and the union representative. Is there any relationship between these roles?
Supervisee: Not really . . .

Silence

   Although I think people probably people come to me more when there are issues because I am an ANUM too.

Supervisor: Is that helpful?
Supervisee: Yeah, I guess.

Silence

   Most of the time it is helpful, but sometimes I think people come to me instead of raising an issue themselves. I shouldn't have to deal with everything.

Organisation

The organisation a supervisee works in shapes the role he or she has and how the role is performed. In order that supervisees are able to fully appreciate and work with the role(s) they hold, they need a comprehensive understanding of the organisation and its impact on role. This is therefore an important component of clinical supervision. A framework for understanding the organisation is provided in the following exercise.

Reflective exercise

The following questions will encourage supervisees to reflect on the broader organisation and the team or unit they work within:

- Why did you choose to work for this particular organisation?
- What keeps you working here?
- What aspects of the organisation do you particularly like?
- What aspects do you not like?
- Are the values of the organisation congruent with your own?
- Would you recommend working at this organisation to others? Why or why not?

The same questions can also be asked about the specific team or unit the supervisees work in.

The supervisees' responses will demonstrate to you the breadth of the context for them, and provide valuable information such as whether they see themselves as an integral part of a larger organisation or tend to define their organisation in relation to their immediate team or unit. This gives important information about the supervisees' context and how they define themselves within their particular organisation.

The next step is to explore the supervisees' definition of organisation with them in more detail, teasing out issues about how the system is structured, such as the governance structures and hierarchies, and the way it functions overall.

Reflective exercise

- Ask supervisees to draw or provide you with the structure of their organisa-tion/team. An organisational map/diagram is usually readily available for each work area and articulates the formal structures. As a supervisor it is useful for you to have a copy of the organisational structure to enhance your knowledge of the formal context in which the supervisees work.
- Next, ask supervisees to draw a diagram of the informal structure of their organisation or team. A basic organisational chart with a genogram overlay-ing it is a really useful strategy as you can identify and highlight relation-ships as well as the structures. These informal diagrams can be really telling as they highlight the organisation and team dynamics, which sometimes do not resemble the formal structures. For example, in some teams the ward clerk, or a particular ANUM rather than the nurse unit manager, maybe the most powerful or influential person in the workplace. All decisions may be 'unofficially' filtered through them first, as the teams knows that without this support decisions will not be made or decisions made not carried through.
- Ask supervisees to identify the significant people within the organisation, to specify the people who are important to them or who influence them in the role they play. This may include mentors, mediators, arbitrators, friends, antagonists and even bullies. Exploration of the team dynamics will also help to identify and highlight particular cliques, subgroupings or alliances. It also provides the basis for identifying conflicts within the team or organisation.
- The usefulness of this information is sometimes questioned. If an individual is in clinical supervision why should so much time be devoted to broader issues? The organisational context of supervisees frames their experiences, how they perceive work and the nature of interactions with staff and patients, and as supervisor it is invaluable information for you to better understand what is influencing and impacting on them. Remember that every issue brought to clinical supervision occurs within the context of the role, organisation and the setting in which it occurs.

Knowledge

Knowledge is a broad area; it is not limited to the formal knowledge that people gain through attending university or participating in workshops. Formal knowledge is important and generally provides the underpinning for professional practice; however, it is not the only source of knowledge and learning. Experience and awareness are also important forms of knowledge. Considering knowledge is an important part of clinical supervision. Under the umbrella of knowledge, supervision can be used to explore what the skill base is and whether the supervisee has what is needed to function effectively in the work environment.

In determining knowledge, the supervisee is likely to explore the following:

* formal learning
* experience
* awareness.

Formal learning

In this section, the supervisor works with supervisees to develop an understanding of their educational background, learning what formal qualifications they have achieved, what workshops they have attended and their participation in other learning environments such as experiential groups or short courses.

Experience

Our experience can be actual practical experience in our clinical area or the experience we have gained through our personal life experiences or in other seemingly unrelated areas. Relevant experience can be gained from a range of contexts. The important thing is how we integrate all these experiences to gain the knowledge required to perform our roles. For example a staff member may have been a volunteer with the Country Fire Authority for a number of years and have applied to work in a high-pressure area such as the emergency department. Past experience and skills gained through having attended some major fires in the past may be very useful in this new context. He or she has demonstrated the ability to function in emergency situations, has been exposed to trauma and is used to working as a team member.

Awareness

This refers to supervisees' awareness of themselves, others and their environment. In discussing this during supervision, the supervisor can gain an understanding about the extent to which supervisees reflect on their practice and the capacity they have to think about the impact they have on their work environment and vice versa.

Accessing the knowledge base

The following questions can assist supervisors to gain this important information:

What is the educational background of the supervisee(s)?
Nursing education has changed greatly over the years and varies from state to state. In order to understand what the supervisee's knowledge base is, the supervisor needs to know more about his or her educational preparation. For example, the extent to which mental health nursing is addressed in undergraduate nursing curricula varies considerably between states but also between universities. It is also generally considered that most courses do not have a strong enough mental health component and consequently, graduates of these programs do not feel confident about their ability to function effectively in this area of practice. The skills and knowledge required for mental health nursing practice are now provided at postgraduate level; however, the current legislation means that postgraduate mental health qualifications are not mandatory for mental health nursing practice in any state or territory with the exception of South Australia.

If you are providing clinical supervision for a nurse working in a mental health setting it would be important to explore the following:

- whether the supervisee has specialist qualifications in mental health nursing
- if not, the size of the mental health nursing component that has been undertaken in the undergraduate program
- the extent to which the supervisee feels educationally prepared to work in the mental health setting
- what other areas he or she is experienced in.

This is really about exploring what the supervisee's professional exposure has been and considering other experiences that could assist in meeting his or her professional goals. For example, some people have had extensive management experience in areas outside of nursing, through other professional experience or through their hobbies or clubs. This is not to be dismissed, as management skills are readily transferable. Working closely with other people and being involved with or accountable for a team means having to deal with the different personalities and conflicts that occur in this environment and is not dissimilar to working as a member of a multidisciplinary team. However, supervisees may not automatically see this connection without the assistance of the supervisor.

Example

During a supervision session, Robert informs you that his unit manager has recently encouraged him to apply for an ANUM position. Robert has a positive relationship with his manager and respects her opinion. He is very interested in the position but has no confidence in his management ability. He tells you that he has settled into this new hospital, enjoys the job and feels at ease with the team he works with and is afraid that he might 'stuff things up' by not performing well in this management role. Through further discussion Robert reveals that he would rather miss out on this opportunity than upset his relationship with the team.

You recall from an earlier session that Robert took over the role of team manager for his brother's basketball team a few years ago. The former manager had left the team following unresolvable conflict between the coach and team manager. The parents of the players were very despondent about the team's viability. A division had developed between supporters of the coach and of the team manager and as a result nobody wanted to step into the team manager role. Robert's brother pleaded with him to take on this position to avoid the team folding. Robert reluctantly agreed.

Robert proved to be very successful in this role. He met with the coach, pledged his support and reinforced the importance that the two work together and deal with any conflict that may emerge between them. He then called a meeting of players and parents. He asked them to remember the purpose of the team and to support their own children and other team members. He asked that any parents with concerns about him or his role discuss the matter with him directly and pay the same respect to the coach. Robert organised some social events to encourage positive interaction between players and parents. The team did not win the grand final that year, but they did have some victories. However, more importantly, the players began to once again enjoy the game and the relationship between parents provided a much more conducive environment for everyone concerned.

Robert's response when you remind him of this is, 'Oh, that was just a kid's basketball team'. As a supervisor you can focus on the skills rather than the setting. Clearly in this example Robert demonstrates high-level skills in management and conflict resolution. He restored morale and possibly prevented the club from folding. It takes some time but you encourage Robert to recognise that he has the skills required to be a successful manager. Robert ultimately decides to apply for the position. He is successful and within weeks he thanks you for 'talking him in to it'. You remind Robert that it was his decision and that you merely encouraged him to look at his skills rather than focusing on his perceived weaknesses.

Reflective exercise

Asking supervisees to draw a time line of their experience can help the supervisor to gain a comprehensive picture of the depth and range of experience a supervisee has.

This involves providing supervisees with a large piece of paper and asking them to record the job, professional roles, hobbies, clubs, etc. they have been involved in. Allow about 20 minutes to complete the task but reassure them they can add to it later if they forgot to mention something.

For the next step, ask supervisees to talk you through each of the entries on the timeline. Do not rush this process: it may run into more than one session. Not only does this process provide you with valuable information, but it also increases the supervisees' awareness of their own skills as they talk about what they have recorded and hopefully become aware of the transferability of these skills.

What knowledge and skills are required for the role(s) the supervisee is in?
In order to develop an adequate understanding of the skills and knowledge required for the role the supervisee is in, it useful to find out as much about the role as you can. Refer to the earlier section on role under context, where role is examined.

Does the supervisee have the knowledge and experience required?
At this point the supervisor asks a number of questions and reflects on the extent to which supervisees have the knowledge and experience required for the role, such as:

- What do they think about their knowledge and experience?
- Do they feel adequately prepared for the role?
- What are your thoughts on how well prepared they are for their role? (This is just a point of reflection for you, not necessarily to share with the supervisee immediately.)
- Where are the gaps?

If either or both of you feel there are some gaps it is important to spend time exploring what they may be and thinking about how they may best be addressed. This can be assisted by the following exercise.

Reflective exercise

If the supervisee you are working with lacks confidence you may want to start working with his or her strengths. This may be harder for the supervisee but it is likely to leave him or her feeling positive rather than reinforcing a negative

Continued

opinion of him- or herself. The supervisee should be aware that both strengths and weaknesses will be explored. If it is possible you may choose to do them concurrently.

Allow approximately 20 minutes with the supervisee helping him or her to identify any parts of the role they avoid, and those they feel least competent and confident in. It is useful to write this down.

Ask the supervisee to apply the same process to the aspects of the role that are most enjoyable and those he or she feels most confident and competent in. It is important to record these also.

An example of some questions that can start the exploration:

Supervisor: I would like you to get yourself in a comfortable position, have a think about the following questions, and write something down that will prompt your memory.

- What is the last thing you tend to do before going home?
  (This question may highlight things left to the last minute because they are not liked or enjoyable parts of the role that are kept to the end of the day as a reward.)
- What part of your role do you never need to remember to do?
  (Again, exploring this will highlight whether it is something the supervisee wants to get over and done or something they cannot wait to do and would never forget.)

Once completed, ask the supervisee to consider what contributes to the avoidance. Is it possible this occurs as a rest of a knowledge gap? Then explore the significance of the parts of the role he or she enjoys, and make the link between enjoyment and other aspects, such as confidence and competence.

It is essential that both areas be explored, as only focusing on the underdeveloped areas or the areas identified as where the supervisee has less confidence could perpetuate and intensify a lack of confidence.

What is the supervisees' self-awareness like? Are they able to identify their strengths and areas of growth?
It will take some time to develop an appreciation for your supervisees' level of awareness. It is through the working relationship over time that you will start to notice how they talk about their own reactions and how they discuss their environment and others working in it. However, you can usually very quickly notice whether they are able to articulate both their strengths and areas of growth. When you speak with them about their work you will notice whether they have any thoughts about how they impact on others and whether their environment is in the picture at all. Promoting awareness is best done through

asking questions and providing the space for supervisees to elaborate. If you say too much and spend a large portion of the time sharing your opinions it could become harder for supervisees to identify how they feel. It is a matter of balance and developing awareness about you as a supervisor.

An example of how to start this exploration

Pay attention to the issues supervisees raise for discussion. When others were involved in the situation you may ask what their responses were, what did they notice and did their responses impact on them at the time?

Relationship

This section focuses on relationships. This includes relationships between supervisee and supervisor, supervisee and patient, supervisee and work colleagues and any other relationships that may impact on the supervisee's work environment.

The primary relationship you will focus on is the one you have with the supervisee. Through this relationship the supervisor can gain some insight into the way in which the supervisee relates to others. For example, if during clinical supervision sessions you find the supervisee to be domineering, always 'right' and reluctant to listen or consider any suggestion you may put forward, you would be likely to reflect on whether he or she adopts the same attitudes and behaviour with colleagues and whether this may explain some of the interpersonal difficulties experienced in the workplace. Often what occurs in clinical supervision is a mirror of what is occurring in other parts of the supervisee's life. With this in mind it is important to pay attention to what you experience within this relationship.

Maintaining boundaries within the relationship

It is crucial that the relationship remains within the framework of clinical supervision. As discussed in Chapter 1, supervision can become confused with other relationships, such as therapy. Even where both parties are clear that clinical supervision is not therapy, the danger that this line could be crossed is ever present. Let us go back to the example of Mary presented in Chapter 1.

Mary desperately wants to have a baby and finds it difficult to care for patients who are terminating a pregnancy, particularly patients like Jennifer who have terminated pregnancies on a number of occasions. As Mary's supervisor you have encouraged her to set goals. Mary has identified that she needs to learn more appropriate ways to come to terms with her own personal issues so she is able to work more therapeutically in these circumstances.

The focus of supervision will clearly be directed towards Mary's role as a nurse in providing effective and therapeutic care for all of her patients irrespective of background and presenting problem. However, Mary is human and finds it difficult (as we all do) to place her work role in a vacuum. During supervision sessions she is inclined to make statements like, 'It's just not fair, these women don't want babies and they keep getting pregnant, I desperately want one and I can't'.

Remember that you are also only human and as a nurse you may well want to respond to her in a therapeutic manner. You may even feel cold and uncaring if you do not do so. You may even move into the role of therapist consciously and subtly. However, doing so would compromise the integrity of the supervision relationship.

Reflective exercise

- What sort of statements from a supervisee might make you feel that the boundary between clinical supervision and therapy is being compromised?
- What sorts of feelings within yourself might sound a warning that you are moving from the role of clinical supervisor to that of therapist?

You may choose to recommend to Mary that she seek therapy, but you need to remain constantly focused on the purpose of your relationship with Mary as a clinical supervisor and encourage her to remain focused on the goals she has set for clinical supervision. Take the time to explain to Mary why you are not going to continue exploring her personal responses in relation to her private life; explain that you have agreed to work with her on her professional life and development.

It can potentially increase a person's vulnerability if you allow them to talk about personal issues in depth, then expect them to switch gears when you meet next and discuss work life. This can be especially problematic if you are providing clinical supervision from within the same organisation. Your supervisee may feel very uncomfortable with you knowing some personal information.

What are the boundaries of the relationship?
It is important to have some clarity about the expectations and limitations within relationships. Boundaries are important because they help promote trust and safety within the relationship. When the boundaries are clear there is less room for problems to arise.

What are the influences on the relationship, positive and negative?
This is about exploring what shapes the relationship. Earlier we discussed how the supervisee relationship is shaped by the supervisee's

motivation. During clinical supervision other relationships of the supervisee will be examined, with consideration of factors that influence the nature of these relationships. For example, supervision may focus on how the supervisee manages his or her workload. If he or she is stressed and feeling unable to cope with the volume of work this is likely to influence engagement with patients and other members of the health care team.

Reflective exercise

Ask the supervisee to focus on a particular relationship within the work context (this may be with either a patient or a colleague) and then do the following:

- Consider in detail and write down the influences shaping that particular relationship.
- Sort these influences into positive or negative, using a white board or cutting and pasting the points.
- Look at what is written overall. After the supervisee has had a chance to read and think about what has been recorded ask if anything is missing that he or she would like to add.
- Assist the supervisee to consider how the negative influences could be managed in order to reduce their impact.
- Similarly examine the positive influences and consider how they could be strengthened.
- Are strong feelings evoked in relation to this person, positive or negative, or does the person remind the supervisee of anyone? These questions are examples of ways to flag the presence of transference and countertransference. Refer to Chapter 5, where these concepts are explained.

Consider your own reactions as a supervisor:

- What kind of responses are evoked in you that may inform you about the relationship, for example a strong negative or positive response? As mentioned above, strong responses are often a sign of transference and countertransference. All strong responses require your immediate attention as a supervisor because they will start to shape how you work with the supervisee. Refer back to the discussion of the psychoanalytic model in Chapter 5.
- What is your capacity to tolerate challenges or alternative views and your ability to hold and articulate your own?

Agreeing to engage in clinical supervision generally means there is some consent by the supervisee to being exposed to challenges or alternative views. Although this may be the case, the reality may be somewhat different. When engaging in a new supervisory relationship you will not be especially aware of the supervisee's capacity in these areas; this will emerge over time. You can, however, work with the supervisee to explore how he or she is with colleagues, which can give you some indication of how he or she may be in clinical supervision. Refer back to Chapter 7 and the section on managing conflicts.

The reflective exercise below includes some questions that might also be useful in increasing your understanding of the supervisee's abilities.

Reflective exercise

Ask the supervisee the following questions, as you consider them appropriate. They do not all need to be asked, they are simply here to provide some ideas. You may like to add some questions of your own.

- Ask the supervisee to identify a situation where he or she felt strongly about something at work but remained silent. In exploring this ensure you develop a full understanding of the situation and the influences that led the supervisee to remain silent.
- Ask the supervisee to identify a situation where he or she felt strongly about something and was able to speak up.

Exploring these first two questions with supervisees will give you some understanding about their capacity to hold their own views and the situations where that capacity is likely to be affected.

- Ask the supervisee if there has been an occasion where he or she has not felt strongly about an issue but became very involved in it. This question is slightly different from the others; it is aimed at understanding whether the supervisee is likely to speak on behalf of others. For example, a colleague has an issue with how a patient is being managed and debriefs with your supervisee. As a result, in the next clinical review the supervisee feels compelled to raise the issues while the colleague, who is also present, remains silent. This is another exercise to increase the supervisee's awareness. Some people tend to take on the spokesperson role but do not become aware of this until they are given the opportunity to explore and reflect upon questions such as these.

Conclusion

This chapter provides a range of techniques to begin a new or to strengthen an existing supervisory relationship. The Hancox/Lynch model includes a framework to provide a degree of structure as a guide for the actual 'doing' of clinical supervision, while still providing sufficient flexibility to be adapted in response to the individual styles of supervisor and supervisee. The introduction of this model is a particular strength of this book. The relevant literature tends to discuss and explain supervision at a theoretical level but falls short of practical tips on how to structure a session and keep the relationship focused on realising its goals. While this is of particular benefit to new supervisors who need a starting point to gain the expertise and confidence as a supervisor, it is also a useful reminder for experienced supervisors, as the supervisory relationship is ever-changing and requires constant monitoring and ongoing reflection. A number of exercises to help you work with your supervisees, increasing your awareness of both your relationship and work environment, have been included.

References

Beinart, H. (2004) Supervision in clinical psychology, theory, practice and perspectives. In: Ian, F. & Linda, S. *Models of Supervision and the Supervisory Relationship and Their Evidence Base*. London: Routledge Taylor and Francis Group, Chapter 3, pp 36–50.

Borwick, I. (2006) Organizational role analysis: Managing strategic change in business settings. In: Newton, J., Long, S. & Sievers, B.K. (eds). *Coaching in Depth The Organizational Role Analysis Approach*. London, New York: Karnac Books.

Hancox, K. & Lynch, L. (2002) *Clinical Supervision for Health Care Professionals. Course Guide*. Melbourne: University of Melbourne and the Centre for Psychiatric Nursing Research and Practice.

Evaluating clinical supervision

Introduction

The key to the sustainability of clinical supervision depends on its champions being able to produce evidence to show that it makes a difference. That evidence will only come through systematic evaluation. The aim of this chapter is to discuss:

- the importance of evaluation
- what evaluation is and how it differs from research
- what should be evaluated
- different types of evaluation
- an overview of methodologies for evaluation
- approaches to measuring impact, including financial, job satisfaction and consumer outcomes.

The importance of evaluation

The effective implementation of clinical supervision requires the investment of considerable resources, both human and monetary. Some of the directly observable costs include:

- training for clinical supervisors and supervisees
- staff time for:
  - ensuring organisational readiness
  - the implementation process
  - marketing and promotion
  - attending training

- providing supervision (if provided internally) or paying for supervision (if provided externally)
- attending supervision
- ongoing monitoring of progress against goals
- maintaining momentum and securing ongoing support.

The associated costs are considerable. In Chapter 3 (where the implementation of clinical supervision in a mental health service in Victoria was described) it was estimated that it cost $A10 000 per month (i.e. $A120 000 per annum) to provide 1 hour of clinical supervision per nurse every 3 weeks. This calculation was based on 144 nurses with an average salary of $A25 per hour. This figure does not take into account any of the additional costs described above, including the cost of the supervisor's time and travel expenses.

Reflective exercise

Think about how the costs listed above might relate to your own organisation.

- How many nurses are employed there? If you do not know this make it a job to find out; you might just be surprised.
- Find an estimate of the average hourly salary rate for nurses.
- Multiply the average hourly rate by the number of nurses in the organisation.
- Multiply by 12 for the annual rate.
- Double the rate in order to account for the supervisor's time (probably an underestimation as clinical supervisors are likely to be more senior than the average nurse).
- Do you need to also factor in any additional expenses such as travelling expenses for both the supervisor and the supervisee (this is a particular issues for rural and regional services)?
- Do you also need to consider training and education costs? How many nurses are in your organisation and how many supervisors are needed? Refer back to Chapter 3. What did your analysis of the organisation tell you about the training and education needs? How many internal or external trainers? Obviously, the costs for internal and external trainers are different and there is always the issue of backfill that needs to be considered.

This provides a rough estimate of the cost of establishment and ongoing costs per month if all nurses were to receive monthly supervision.

It would be difficult to secure that level of funding at the best of times, however, the economically constrained environment we are all working in makes this all the more difficult. No organisation is likely to invest even a proportion of that money without considerable confidence that the investment will be justified. Even if the support of management is secured, factors like a further economic downturn or changes within management can result in support previously given being withdrawn. Safety will only come with strong evidence of cost-effectiveness.

The champions of clinical supervision will argue that it is not all about money, no argument here! But at the end of the day those responsible for managing the health service budget will need to be convinced substantially on economic grounds. This is not to suggest that economic benefits should be the exclusive focus of evaluation. Those who drive the clinical supervision agenda will have many questions about effectiveness.

Reflective exercise

- What do you think the effective introduction of clinical supervision would look like?
- What outcomes do you believe would convince you that clinical supervision is worth maintaining?
- How would you be able to tell if these outcomes had been achieved?
- Ask some of your key stakeholders for their views. These key stakeholders are likely to be the ones you identified in Chapter 3 as those individuals who are important to your overall strategy.

The answers to these questions will give you some ideas as to how you might go about evaluating the effectiveness of clinical supervision. Some of your outcomes might readily lend themselves to evaluation, e.g. reduced staff turnover, while others may be more difficult, e.g. more satisfied staff, improvement in team or group dynamics. Because evaluation involves working with people, with a complex array of attitudes and opinions, and the many factors that influence them, some of the answers we consider most valuable can be the most difficult to discover.

This chapter is not intended as a comprehensive guide to evaluation. There are many high-quality books on this topic. Nor does it profess to have all of the answers. The primary aim is to encourage you to consider the importance of evaluation and the approaches you might use in evaluating the effectiveness of clinical supervision that reflect the values of the organisation you work for.

Distinguishing between research and evaluation

The same methods of data collection and analysis are often used in both research and evaluation, which can lead to confusion between the two. However, despite some important similarities between the two there are some significant differences. Research involves a systematic inquiry with the aim of validating existing knowledge and/or creating new knowledge. A specific aim of research is to use the findings to make assumptions, which can be applied or generalised to other settings. Evaluation may (and should) be equally rigorous in its approach but it is designed to meet specific local needs to determine if a specific program or initiative is effective within that specific context.

For example, both research and evaluation may be concerned with the number of nurses who elect to receive clinical supervision and the extent to which they find it valuable. In terms of numbers or percentages, the figures will be important knowledge for the researcher and would be reported as results of the study. The evaluator will also want to know the rate of uptake but will generally judge (or evaluate) this against a preconceived set of expectations. Let us say 10% of nurses engage in clinical supervision. In the case of research, this figure will be presented. It is also likely that theoretical assumptions about clinical supervision will be attempted. Data on the demographic characteristics of the nurses who became involved may be compared to those who did not to determine the impact of factors such as age, gender and years of experience in nursing. This information will be used to make theoretical assumptions, for example that older, more experienced females are more likely to embrace the notion of clinical supervision. A similar study could be undertaken in another setting to see if the same characteristics apply. Publication is an important end product of research. The published information becomes available to interested parties (researchers, evaluators, managers and clinicians) as a contribution to knowledge in this area.

The evaluator, on the other hand, is interested in knowing whether or not the implementation of clinical supervision worked. The reaction to a 10% uptake would be influenced by a preconceived idea of what should be achieved. If the expectation was for 50% then the team would consider that this initiative was not successful, whereas if they expected only 5% (albeit unlikely) they would be pleased with these results. The success or failure is of interest to the team primarily as it relates to their specific organisation – did it work or didn't it? So even when the same method is used, the reason for the study and its intended applications are generally different.

What should be evaluated?

In deciding what needs to be evaluated, the starting point must be: what do you want to know? And what do you need to convince management that clinical supervision is worth supporting?

If you completed the exercise in the first section, you should already be on the way to answering the first question. Each health care organisation is unique, as are the people who champion the cause of clinical supervision, and therefore the exact focus of your evaluation is not likely to be the same as that of any other organisation. However, we offer the following suggestions for your consideration (you may well have already thought of many of them).

The process

- Has the implementation process been successful?
- What unexpected issues have emerged? How have these been overcome?
- What further work needs to be done (refer back to the Lynch model of implementation described in Chapter 3)?
- Have the education and training provided been successful? Is any more required?

Supervisee perceptions

- What is the uptake of clinical supervision?
- Why have some nurses chosen not to participate?
- Do those who are participating think it is a good thing? What specific benefits do supervisees gain from it?
- Are supervisees able to leave the workplace for supervision without repercussions or barriers?

Supervisor perceptions

- Do supervisors feel competent and confident to perform this role?
- Have any legal or ethical issues emerged?
- Are supervisors satisfied with the level of supervisee attendance and preparation?
- Are supervisors able to manage the supervisory role within their existing workload (a particularly important issue as supervisors are likely to provide clinical supervision for more than one nurse)?
- Do supervisors need any additional support?

Management perspectives

- Do management support this initiative? If so, how strong is their support?
- Are management likely to (continue to) support this initiative in the future?
- What do management perceive as the impact on the individual unit or team and the broader organisation following the introduction of clinical supervision?
- Have management observed any tangible, beneficial outcomes to date?

Economic benefits

These are evidenced by observable improvements in areas such as reduction in:

- sick leave
- stress leave or work cover
- critical incidents
- staff turnover.

Practice benefits

- Is there any noticeable difference in the practice for nurses receiving clinical supervision?
- Has patient care improved?
- Has patient satisfaction increased?

Feel free to add other considerations to this list. We do not assume for a moment that this is exhaustive.

Different types of evaluation

Posavac & Carey (2007) identify four main approaches to evaluation:

- evaluating need
- evaluating the process
- evaluating the outcomes
- evaluating efficiency.

A brief description of each is presented here.

Evaluating need

It is likely you are familiar with the term 'needs analysis', which effectively means the assessment of needs. Health care organisations will not embark on the implementation of clinical supervision because it seems like a good idea, but rather because it presents a potential solution to a currently unmet need. Through conducting a needs analysis, the lack of support and professional development opportunities for nurses may be identified. Before deciding on clinical supervision, a number of other possible approaches are likely to be considered. The Lynch model is stage 1, where clinical supervision is considered amongst a number of possible initiatives to determine whether it will meet the desired goals of the organisation (see Chapter 3).

Evaluating the process

Determining the success or otherwise of clinical supervision is not simply a matter of giving it a go and finding out later whether or not it has worked. It is important to gather information about the actual process of implementation itself. This involves determining what is required to maximise the chances of success. During the implementation process itself, the team must be mindful about whether the process is occurring according to plan and whether clinical supervision is in fact meeting the needs of the organisation as previously anticipated. It involves recognition of the influences that support the initiative and those that potentially undermine its effectiveness. The Lynch model (particularly stages 2–5) provides a useful guide to evaluating the process of implementing clinical supervision.

Process evaluation can be quite challenging. Once a team has identified an initiative they think will be positive for the organisation, there is a tendency to want to get in and make it happen. However, if it proves to be successful or otherwise it is important to know what contributed to the success or failure. It also allows the time to recognise unexpected outcomes and deal with them as they emerge. Initiatives are rarely implemented exactly as planned and clinical supervision will be no exception. A thorough and comprehensive evaluation of the process will provide a solid basis from which clinical supervision could be implemented elsewhere in the organisation, or indeed in other organisations grappling with the same underlying issues.

Evaluating the outcomes

As clinical supervision was implemented to address a specific need within the organisation, it is important to know whether or not it has achieved the desired effect. For example, are nurses engaging in clinical supervision? Do they feel more confident and competent in their role as a result? Does management identify positive change? Has an improvement in patient care been observed?

Some methods that might be used to obtaining this information will be outlined in the next section; however, it is important to be mindful of the difficulties in determining whether changes have occurred as a direct result of the introduction of clinical supervision. Research and evaluation involving humans is particularly complex due to the dynamic interactions that occur between people themselves, and between people and the broader environment in which the initiative takes place. An evaluation may demonstrate positive outcomes following the implementation of clinical supervision, but how can we be confident that these outcomes are the result of clinical supervision? The findings could be the result of other factors not accounted for in the evaluation, such as the appointment of a new unit manger with a different approach or other staffing changes resulting in a different dynamic within the work environment. Indeed, the intervention itself can result in changes. Nurses may feel more positive because management is responding to their needs and it may be that any other intervention may have been equally effective.

This does not mean that evaluation is not effective or not worth the trouble. However, it suggests that more effective evaluation requires multiple methods (discussed further below) to enhance confidence that clinical supervision, and not something else, has influenced the outcomes. For example, survey results may show improved staff morale. This could be followed up by interviews with staff to find out more about why this has occurred. Interviews would provide the opportunity for staff to describe why they feel more positive about their work environment, with specific questions about how clinical supervision may have contributed.

Evaluating efficiency

Matters of finance come into play with any initiative. As demonstrated in Chapter 3, clinical supervision can be a costly initiative and managers will want to be confident that the money is well spent. Any initiative that can demonstrate economic benefits to the organisation, or at least be cost neutral, will have a far greater chance of being sustained. The ability to demonstrate cost-effectiveness should therefore be built into any evaluation of clinical supervision. This could include demonstrating a decrease in staff turnover, sick leave or critical incidents. Again it is difficult to show a direct relationship between clinical supervision and this sort of change, but combined with other forms of evaluation it may contribute to a stronger argument in support of clinical supervision.

An overview of methodologies for evaluation

Once you are clear about what it is important to know, consideration can be given to identifying the best approaches to ensure you find the best possible answers to your question. We used the term 'approaches' because it is unlikely you will find one method to assist in answering all of these questions.

The methods that can be used for evaluation are:

- qualitative
- quantitative
- cost–benefit analysis.

Qualitative methods

As the name suggests, qualitative methods emphasise the quality or depth of information rather than the amount (quantity). The primary aim of qualitative methods is to interpret and understand human social phenomena through descriptive analyses that focus on the discovery and articulation of participants' attitudes, opinions and feelings. The focus is on the individual's unique experience rather than a broader application that can be transferred to other people or groups.

Because of the intensive nature of data collection, usually a relatively small number of participants can be included. This means that the outcomes cannot be generalised to the population of interest. The value of qualitative methods is often criticised for its inability to provide reliable information about specific populations. However, this is not the aim of qualitative methods, where the focus is on uniqueness and individuality.

There are two main techniques for the collection of qualitative data, namely:

- in-depth interviews (individual and focus group)
- observation (participant and non-participant).

In-depth individual interviews

In-depth individual interviews are a popular method for the collection of qualitative data. These interviews are often described as a form of conversation. Developing a conversational tone is important because it puts the participant at ease and therefore creates the conditions for the participant to freely and openly discuss insights, opinions and experiences. In-depth interviews are generally conducted face-to-face in order to facilitate open communication. However, interviews are sometimes conducted by telephone when in-person interviews are not possible (for example, over geographical distances).

Legard *et al.* (2004) identify six main stages of the in-depth interview:

(1) The arrival, where trust and rapport are established.
(2) Introduction of the topic. At this stage a clear description of the nature and purpose is provided. Issues relating to confidentiality should be raised and permission to tape the interview (if required) should be obtained at this time.
(3) Beginning the interview. This involves seeking factual background information to assist with the formulation of questions, for example, 'What made you decide to seek clinical supervision?' If the participant responds that she was told by her manager, the types of questions to follow are likely to be different than if she responded that she has always wanted to have clinical supervision so that as soon as the opportunity came up she was there!
(4) During the interview. This is the stage where the interviewee is guided through the main topics the interviewer seeks to cover. However, equally important, the interviewer will respond to issues raised by the participant.
(5) Ending the interview. Towards the end of the interview, the interviewer will begin the wind-up process, giving the interviewee the

opportunity to provide further comments or clarification. It is important to ensure that the interviewee is not left with any unexpressed feelings or issues.

(6)   After the interview. This is the time to thank interviewees for their contribution and to provide reassurance regarding confidentiality. This is particularly important if interviewees raise issues of a personal or sensitive nature, or disclose names of people or organisations.

Because in-depth interviews resemble conversation, it is sometimes assumed that they are easy to conduct. In fact, the reverse is true. There is great skill involved in conducting a fruitful and productive interview to produce the depth and type of information sought. The interviewer must be able to respond to the interviewee, asking probing questions to illicit further information, whilst at the same time ensuring that the interview retains some focus. In short, interviewers need to be flexible but structured naturalistic in-depth interviewers.

Focus groups

Focus groups, as the name implies, involve interviewing a number of people (usually between six and ten) at the same time. One obvious advantage of focus groups is the opportunity to interview more people than would be possible in an individual situation. Ten people can be interviewed in a focus group much more easily than interviewing 10 people individually. However, this should not be a major consideration. Individual interviews and focus groups serve different purposes in much the same way as individual and group supervisions do (see Chapter 4). The primary advantage of focus groups is the interaction and discussion that occurs. Ideas can be bounced off the different participants, with members being able to respond to issues raised by others that they might not have considered themselves.

There are also disadvantages to focus groups. Less time is available for each participant to contribute because they share the time with other people. More vocal and assertive members may dominate the discussion, leaving less opportunity for quieter people to have their say (Kevern & Webb, 2001; McHugh & Thoms, 2001). Under these circumstances it is difficult to determine the extent to which the data collected are representative of the group as a whole rather than of a small number of dominant members. It can also be difficult to organise focus groups for a time and place when all the participants can be there (Reed, 2005).

There are times when focus groups should definitely not be used, for example when there are power differentials between participants, because the less powerful members may not feel comfortable in expressing views in opposition to those from greater positions of power (Happell, 2007).

Finch & Lewis (2004) identify five major stages of a focus group:

(1) Scene setting and ground rules. Confidentiality is an important consideration in focus groups, particularly when the members know each other socially or through work. There needs to be a shared commitment that information disclosed within the group must not be divulged outside of the group.
(2) Individual introductions. This is particularly important where the interviewees do not know one another. However, even when they do, introductions provide the opportunity for the interviewer to know more about the group, and of course for the group to know more about the interviewer.
(3) The opening topic.
(4) Discussion.
(5) Ending the discussion. Essentially, this is similar to the ending process for the individual interview.

Preparing for the interview

Whether you choose an individual or focus group approach, it is important that you are well prepared for the interview. Although successful interviews might adopt a conversational approach, they differ from social interactions in that they have a specific purpose. While you want to encourage the participant(s) to express their own views and opinions, you want to be sure they are relevant to your area of interest. For example, if you choose to conduct focus groups to determine the nurses' responses to the introduction of clinical supervision, you should not have preconceived ideas of what they will tell you (such as 'Clinical supervision is fantastic, we love it'), but equally you do not want the conversation to divert to the broader problems of the organisation (for example, 'If we could only get rid of the director of nursing and get more staff everything would be fine').

In order to ensure that the interview addresses the specific topics of interest, the interviewer should develop a list or schedule of questions to act as a guide for the interview.

Developing the interview guide

The guide should be developed with the input of the evaluation team. Careful consideration must be given to the type of information that will help to determine if clinical supervision has been successfully implemented, the positive and negative aspects as perceived by the stakeholders, and any specific issues that need to be addressed. The guide should further be informed by referring to the literature, describing what has already been conducted in the area.

The information sought in interviews will probably vary depending on the stakeholder group (i.e. managers, supervisors, supervisees), and therefore the guide should be tailored to reflect this. For example, managers may be more interested in the impact on the efficiency of the organisation, supervisors on their readiness for and confidence in the role, while supervisees might be more concerned with the impact of clinical supervision on their ability to provide care for people with complex needs.

Taking the example of supervisees, the evaluation team may decide that the following information would be useful:

- How easily have supervisees been able to access clinical supervision? This question may then give rise to the following issues:
  - Have there been problems in finding an available supervisor the supervisees can work with?
  - Has there been difficulty in being released from the unit or team to attend sessions?
  - Have supervisees found it personally difficult to leave the unit or team to attend sessions? That is, do they feel guilty about leaving their work for others to do?

When incorporating these issues into the interview guide, it is important not to lead the participant(s) (either consciously or unconsciously) to provide the answers you may be hoping or expecting to hear. For example, if you anticipate that supervisees have had difficulty being released from their clinical load you might be tempted to ask 'What problems have you experienced in being permitted to attend clinical supervision?' Such a question automatically implies: (1) there is a problem and (2) the responsibility lies with management. This assumption may be incorrect, but even if it is accurate, the question has led the participants to a particular way of thinking and they are now focusing on that aspect of the situation. In doing so, they may not address other barriers, such as their personal reluctance to leave the unit because they feel they are letting the team down.

To allow for a broader range of issues and opinions to be addressed, the question might be better stated as 'Please describe any factors that make it easy or difficult for you to attend clinical supervision sessions.' By reframing the question in this way there is no assumption that a problem exists but the opportunity is there for participants to talk about the factors that might enhance attendance (supportive unit manager/team leader, support from peers who willingly take responsibility for the nurse's clinical load during this time), as well as those that detract (lack of support from management and colleagues). Furthermore, it provides scope for broader systemic issues (lack of experienced staff, admission of patients with high acuity levels) or problems with the supervisor (cancels appointments at short notice, is not prepared, does not seem interested) to be addressed.

The evaluation team is often very keen and enthusiastic to get out there and start asking questions, but while a more considered approach may take longer, it is likely to reap rewards by producing deeper and more accurate information.

In the interview situation itself it is important that the guide be seen as just that, a guide. It is very unlikely that the evaluation team will consider all areas of interest and concern to the participants and they may well raise issues not previously considered by team members. Indeed, one of the major advantages of qualitative research is that it provides sufficient flexibility for the participants' perspective to be revealed. If a prescriptive interview guide is used then this advantage will be lost. The structure of the interviews needs to be sufficiently loose to give participants the space and opportunity to air any issues they feel are relevant. The guide should therefore be used only to ensure that specific information is obtained and that there is a degree of consistency between the series of interviews. The interviewer should not read from it but rather refer to it at various stages to ensure that essential information is captured. The scope to move away from the predetermined information should be present and it should be made obvious to participants that it is their knowledge and opinions that constitute the primary focus of the interviews.

Interviews that are based on a broad interview guide in this manner are generally referred to as semi-structured interviews, which distinguishes this approach from unstructured interviews (with little or no specific focus) or structured interviews (where the participant is asked to respond to a series of preset questions).

Types of questions

During the interview process two main types of questions are generally used: open and closed.

Closed questions are designed to elicit specific and factual answers, for example:

- How long have you worked in this organisation?
- What is your current position?
- What are your qualifications?

Participants will generally answer these questions with specific information, for example 10 years; associate nurse unit manager; Bachelor of Nursing, Postgraduate Diploma in Critical Care Nursing.

Open questions are designed to elicit views, opinions and experiences. They are therefore phrased in a way that encourages participants to consider the issue in depth and respond with more detail than they would for a closed question. Examples of open questions are:

- Please describe any changes to your ability to practice as a nurse as the result of receiving clinical supervision.
- How do you consider (if at all) that clinical supervision has been of benefit to you?

- What do you see as the major limitations (if any) to clinical supervision?

You will note the inclusion of 'if at all' or 'if any' as part of the question. This is to avoid leading the participant into thinking that they should be able to identify benefits or limitations and that the interviewer is expecting this.

Tips for a successful interview

As discussed above, a successful interview should be as conversational as possible to allow people to openly discuss their thoughts and opinions, but with sufficient structure to ensure the topics of interest are addressed. Interviewing requires significant skill and experience. If the information is worth getting then do not make the mistake of picking just anyone to ask the questions. The following tips may be helpful in making sure the interviews are as successful as possible:

- Choose a location where the participant(s) will feel comfortable and which is likely to be free of interruptions.
- Ensure a comfortable setting.
- Make sure you are familiar with the contents of the interview guide. Keep the guide close enough that you are able to make quick reference without disrupting the flow of the interview.
- Ask questions clearly and clarify as necessary. You should be clear about the intent and purpose of the questions you are asking but the participants may not be.
- Be comfortable with silence. Allow participants time to think about the questions and their responses to them. Inexperienced interviewers often interrupt this process because they interpret silence as uncertainty or lack of interest in the questions. Relax and give thinking time.

Participant and non-participant observation

As a method of research and evaluation, observation is used to study and understand the dynamics of a situation as it occurs. While interviews produce valuable data, for that period of time the interviewee is removed from the phenomena of interest, meaning that the information imparted reflects attitudes and opinions. Observation provides the opportunity to see what is actually happening and to examine such factors as relationships between people.

It is important to note that observation is not a casual or haphazard process of 'taking a look'. The observer generally has a clear idea of the type of activities he or she wishes to observe and has developed a system to record these observations. The importance of this level of preparation is demonstrated in the following example.

Reflective exercise

Think about one of your favourite movies that you have watched more than once. Discuss it with others and consider:

- The aspects of the movie that initially appealed to you.
- How your views changed after watching it for the second or third time.
- Were there important or interesting parts to the movie that you did not notice the first time?
- Have your friends had different views or noticed different things of interest in the movie?

When people watch movies, particularly those they find especially interesting or entertaining, they tend to become absorbed. Often they focus on some aspects at the expense of others. For example, they become so involved in the relationship between the two main characters they may not see, or fully appreciate, the underlying hostility between the female lead and her mother. They may also be so curious with wanting to know what happens next that some of the immediate details are be overlooked.

In the case of movies, we can watch them as many times as we like, thus giving us the opportunity to pick up on details previously missed. Observation does not come with the same luxury. Because the observer cannot hit the replay button, he or she must get the most out of one opportunity.

The two main types of observation are participant and non-participant. Both have their respective advantages and disadvantages, and are briefly discussed here.

Participant observation

As the name suggests, this form of observation involves becoming part of and involved in the culture of the people and situations being observed. Participant observation usually takes place over a considerable time period to allow the observer to establish rapport and gain the confidence of the study population. In effect, the observer must become part of the environment.

The high level of immersion of the observer within the study environment is a significant advantage of participant observation; the observer is likely to witness things that would not emerge in an interview situation. However, this is potentially also a major disadvantage. In becoming such a part of the situation, the observer may lose the 'big picture'; she or he may become so much a part of it that the role of participant overshadows that of observer, and the focus becomes doing rather than seeing. In the process of becoming part of the group, the observer has limited opportunity to record field notes and therefore important data may be lost. Participant observation is also expensive and time-consuming.

Non-participant observation
This involves the observer remaining separate to or detached from the study environment and observing what happens without involvement. The idea is to be like a hidden camera. In being detached, the observer is less likely to be directly influenced by the people or environment, and therefore is more able to be objective.

The issue of presumed objectivity also represents a potential disadvantage to this approach. The fact that observation takes place at a distance and without direct involvement means that the observer is likely to interpret and make sense of what is seen according to his or her own values and beliefs without a comprehensive understanding of what the actions or behaviours may mean to those directly involved.

Another major disadvantage is that the presence of the observer alters the actions and behaviours of those being observed. Think about your own experiences when others are watching you and taking particular note of what you do. Your response may reflect a level of anxiety, where you find it more difficult to do the things you would normally do as a matter of course because you are concerned with how you appear to be. You may also be on your best behaviour, trying to impress the observer that you are skilled and competent, or considerate and friendly. The impact of this disadvantage can be minimised by spending lengthy periods in the study environment in order that people become used to being observed, and relax and behave more naturally. However, once again this becomes an expensive and time-consuming process.

Relevance to clinical supervision
The principles of non-participant observation are often utilised as a training technique, particularly in developing the skills required of a supervisor. This involves watching a clinical supervision interaction and providing feedback to the supervisor about issues such as communication style, body language, ability to pick up on key points, etc. It can also be used with supervisees, for example to consider their response to supervisor suggestions or the extent to which they become engaged with the process.

In some instances the supervisors and supervisees themselves may take a participant observer role by feeding back their responses to one another. However, the difficulty of being actively involved in the supervision process whilst remaining detached enough to evaluate the process itself presents a level of difficulty that may not be easily overcome.

Due to the time and expense involved in both forms of observation, and the likely impact of the observer on the interactions, this is not likely to be widely used as an approach to evaluation.

Quantitative research

By definition, quantitative research is concerned with quantity, that is with measuring or counting the variables of interest. The primary aim of quantitative research is to measure, count or classify human phenomena, actions or characteristics using numerical and statistical techniques.

A significant difference between qualitative and quantitative methods is that the latter can be used to make generalisations about larger groups or populations, or to determine relationships between factors and variables, for example the degree to which one factor or characteristic influences or determines another. The primary disadvantage of quantitative methods is that in order to secure an adequate number of responses from a large population, there are limitations to the number of questions that can be asked or the number of alterative responses that can be offered. Researchers can therefore achieve quantity but are limited in the degree of quality (i.e. depth of opinion or experience).

Types of quantitative methods used in evaluation

There are far too many quantitative methods to be fairly addressed in this chapter. However, you may well be familiar with the following:

- randomised controlled trial (RCT)
- quasi-experimental design
- systematic review
- meta-analysis
- survey research.

The methods most likely to be used to evaluate the implementation of clinical supervision are survey research and quasi-experimental designs. This is not to suggest that other approaches might not also be useful, but given the limitations of space, surveys and quasi-experimental approaches will receive the primary focus.

Survey research

Surveying refers to the process of collecting data from a group of people who are considered to represent a larger population. Data are collected through the use of a suitable instrument or tool comprising a number of questions, which may be closed or open ended (discussed below). Surveys may be researcher-administered or self-administered and may be completed face-to-face, by telephone, via the internet or via post.

Closed questions refer to those where respondents are required to make a choice based on the information provided to them. In some cases this is simple, for example when asked one's gender, the vast majority of us can simply answer male or female. However, closed questions are often used to measure values or opinions that do not lend themselves so easily to categorisation. Take, for example, the importance of the right of an individual to choose his or her own clinical supervisor. How might this be measured with a quantitative approach?

Generally, this type of variable would be measured with the use of a Likert scale. This requires participants to assign a numerical value according to how strongly they agree with or feel about a particular issue or phenomena. In answering the question posed above, the person would be required to respond with a number usually ranging from 1 to 7 (although variations on this can also be used). The lower numbers usually refer to a level of disagreement and the higher numbers to a level of agreement. Note the following example of a 7-point Likert scale:

(1)   very strongly disagree
(2)   strongly disagree
(3)   disagree
(4)   neither agree or disagree/uncertain
(5)   agree
(6)   strongly agree
(7)   very strongly agree

In answering the question the respondent considers how strongly he or she feels about the right to free speech. This approach is more sensitive to the degree of opinion than a simple yes/no response would be.

A major advantage of the Likert scale approach is the quick response time, allowing a number of questions to be addressed in a relatively short time frame. The major disadvantage is that the participant's views and opinions are automatically limited by the questions asked. In the example above the participant may indicate how important the right to choose one's supervisor is, but there is no room to explore the issue more broadly. For example, why choice is or is not important cannot be explored unless additional questions are asked.

As Likert scales produce numerical data, analysis is a relatively straightforward and expedient process.

The advantages and disadvantages of open-ended questions are generally the opposite to those of closed questions. While the open question provides more opportunity for participants to express their views and opinions, the data produced need to be coded before entry and analysis. Coding data is generally a very time-consuming process and therefore tends to limit the number and complexity of questions asked.

Table 9.1 Advantages and disadvantages of open and closed questions.

	Advantages	Disadvantages
Closed	• Easy and quick to answer (participants more likely to complete the questions) • Participants can respond to options rather than thinking up an answer • Socially less desirable responses can be included as an option (participants may be more likely to respond to such an option than to initiate it) • Responses are usually clear and complete • Data are easy to standardise, code and analyse • Suitable for either self-completion or completion with researcher help	• Depend on participants understanding what is required of them and the concept of a preference or rating scale • Participants may just guess or tick any response at random • Participants or researchers may make errors (e.g. tick the wrong box by mistake) • Do not allow participants to expand on their responses or offer alternative views
Open	• Allow participants to respond based on views and opinions • Capture responses, feelings and ideas that researchers may not have thought of • Participants may write as much or as little as they wish	• Take longer to complete (which can dissuade people from responding) • Responses can be extremely laborious (and expensive) to analyse – coding and interpretation needed • If handwriting is not clear data are lost • Rely on participants wanting to be expressive and having writing skills • Reponses are often superficial, not providing the depth the evaluation team are seeking

The advantages and disadvantages of both open and closed questions are presented in Table 9.1.

Surveys and questionnaires

Surveys and questionnaires are popular forms of data collection because they are relatively easy to administer, score, analyse and interpret, and potentially provide data from a large number of participants. Surveys and questionnaires can be used as the main method of data collection or they can be combined with other quantitative and qualitative techniques.

People often make the mistake of thinking that the construction and design of a questionnaire is simply a matter of producing a list of interesting and relevant questions. On the contrary, Boynton & Greenhalgh (2004) state:

*Anybody can write down a list of questions and photocopy it, but produc-
ing worthwhile and generalisable data from questionnaires needs careful
planning and imaginative design . . . Inappropriate instruments and lack
of rigour inevitably lead to poor quality data, misleading conclusions,
and woolly recommendations.* (p. 1312)

Designing a valid and reliable questionnaire

As is the case for all forms of research, this process should begin with
a clear understanding of the information that will assist you to answer
your research questions. It is important to appreciate the range of possible responses in order to ensure that the right questions are asked.
While the evaluation team itself is likely to make a significant contribution in terms of knowledge and ideas, it is not likely that they will
consider all possibilities.

A deeper breadth of information can be gained from additional
sources, including a literature and expert opinion. If these areas are
found to be insufficient a qualitative exploratory approach may be used
to ensure that the views and opinions of multiple stakeholders are
reflected in the final instrument.

It is also important that the evaluation questions can be adapted for
a questionnaire. Researchers and evaluators often choose open-ended
questions with plenty of blank space on the form and are surprised
when they receive only 10–15-word responses to a question such as
'How has engagement with clinical supervision altered your clinical
practice?' As a rule of thumb participants have nowhere near the same
level of interest in the study as the team itself, and therefore do not
devote the time and attention that might be hoped or planned for.

Evaluation teams are often enthusiastic about answering every
possible question that could provide important information about the
implementation of clinical supervision, and therefore want to develop
their own questionnaire. Developing a new questionnaire is generally
a time-consuming process. Not only do you need to develop the questions themselves, but a pilot study and initial data analysis are also
necessary to ensure that the instrument is valid and reliable. It is therefore advisable to identify and critique previously validated and published questionnaires. Not only will this save considerable time, but it
also provides a stronger baseline to compare your findings with others
using the same questionnaire. If you are planning to publish your findings in a nursing or health care journal, using a previously validated
and preferably well-known tool is useful.

However, the aim of evaluating clinical supervision is to answer
specific questions about its value and usefulness. If you cannot find a
questionnaire that addresses this, the fact that it is validated and widely
used will not compensate for its lack of relevance to your study. Sometimes evaluation teams use an existing questionnaire as a basis and
adapt it by adding and/or deleting questions or by altering the wording

of certain questions. This is likely to make the questionnaire more relevant but any alterations mean that the validity and reliability of the questionnaire must be determined anew.

The way in which questionnaires are designed and presented is also important. Well-presented and clearly structured questionnaires are more likely to be completed than those lacking clarity and structure. Table 9.2 presents some handy tips for the preparation of questionnaires.

Using questionnaires for clinical supervision research

There could be several uses for questionnaires in clinical supervision research. Firstly, they could be used to determine satisfaction with the initiative in a descriptive sense. This type of questionnaire might ask a combination of open and closed questions seeking participant opinions about whether clinical supervision:

- is useful
- is enjoyable
- is a good use of the time invested in it
- improves work satisfaction
- improves nursing practice.

Further questions could explore whether:

- nurses are able to leave the unit to engage in clinical supervision
- clinical supervision is supported by management
- the clinical supervisor is reliable
- the clinical supervisee is reliable.

As an alternative or adjunct to a descriptive survey, the team may use a rating scale or series of rating scales to measure specific factors that might influence nursing work, such as job satisfaction, stress, burnout and nursing care. Examples of such scales are:

- Maslach's burnout inventory (Maslach & Jackson, 1986)
- Minnesota Satisfaction Questionnaire (Weiss et al., 1967)
- Manchester Clinical Supervision Survey (Winstanley, 2000).

Rating scales are generally used to determine change over a period of time. In the case of clinical supervision, the scales are administered prior to commencement (known as pre-test or baseline data) and after one or more specific time periods, e.g. 6 months, 12 months or 2 years (known as post-test data). Statistical data analysis is then used to determine if clinical supervision is effective by comparing the results from the two time points, that is positive changes in scores may provide evidence for the effectiveness of clinical supervision.

It is important to note that findings from this type of evaluation would need to be interpreted with caution. Nurses and the health care environments they work in are complex and dynamic. Changes on

Table 9.2 Designing questionnaires (Boynton & Greenhalgh, 2004).

Section	Quality criterion
Title	Should be simple and clear Should give a concise but accurate description of the focus of the evaluation
Introductory letter or information sheet	Must provide a succinct outline of the evaluation and its overall purpose Should include an estimation of the time it should take to complete the questionnaire The way in which the anonymity and confidentiality of participants will be protected must be described It is important to emphasise that completion of the questionnaire is completely voluntary and that participants can change their minds even after beginning to complete the questionnaire without needing to provide a reason The contact details of the members of the evaluation team who can provide further information must be clearly recorded Postage-paid envelopes addressed to the researcher should be included with postal questionnaires
Overall layout	The font must be large enough, recommend 12 point with 10 point as a minimum The questionnaire should look attractive. Graphics, illustrations and colour may help with this but it is important to ensure that the finished product looks professional. The questions rather than the extras should be the focus Ensure that pages are numbered and stapled securely in the right order Clear and concise instructions on how to complete each item must be provided with examples given where necessary
Demographic information	Ensure that you have all the information necessary for developing a profile of the participants, e.g. age, gender, length of nursing experience Do not include misleading or superfluous questions, for example marital status is often included as a standard question, even where this is not likely to be relevant, such as in evaluating clinical supervision Ensure questions are not offensive or otherwise inappropriate, giving consideration to gender, culture and ethnicity
Measures (main body of questionnaire)	Ensure measures are valid and reliable Remove unnecessary or repetitive questions Make sure the questionnaire is not too long Give careful consideration to the order of questions as this could influence responses or reduce participation rates, for example sensitive or personal questions should be placed towards the end
Closing comments	A clear statement to mark the end of the questionnaire should be included The participants should be thanked for their time and involvement
Accompanying materials	If the questionnaire is to be returned by post, a stamped addressed envelope (with return address on it) should be included

rating scales could be the result of a number of influencing factors, for example change in management, change in staffing profile or improvements to the physical environment such as the refurbishment of the unit.

To make the research more rigorous, sometimes other units or teams of nurses who are not receiving clinical supervision are given the same questionnaires over the same time period. This is known as a control group, and the group receiving clinical supervision is the experimental group. Comparing the findings from the two groups using statistical analysis provides some basis for assuming that the differences between the two groups after the introduction of clinical supervision is the result of this initiative, providing of course that the two groups were essentially similar at the pre-test stage.

The inclusion of a control group increases the strength of the research but falls short of proving or demonstrating cause and effect. Even if clear differences are found at the post-test stage, with more positive outcomes for the experimental group, the cause could be something other than clinical supervision. The differences could be the result of the Hawthorn effect, which means that the findings reflect the research process itself rather than the intervention, that is the nurses may be experiencing less burnout and feeling more satisfied with their work environment because:

- management is prepared to commit funds to support nursing
- the presence of the evaluation team makes them feel they are receiving special treatment
- they have the opportunity to leave the ward or team for a specified period of time.

You may ask, if the results are positive, does it really matter whether or not clinical supervision is the primary influencing factor, the Hawthorn effect will do just nicely? Unfortunately, the Hawthorn effect is usually short term. To be more confident that positive outcomes are the result of clinical supervision, the evaluation should be extended over a longer period of time. The Hawthorn effect may be an explanation for changes noted after 6 months, but would be much less likely to be a major influence after a year and less likely still after 2 years. While a longer duration of the evaluation means the findings are more likely to be an accurate measure of the impact of clinical supervision, this will require additional resources, particularly time and money, which tend to be finite in health care organisations.

Sampling method

Sampling refers to the process used to select participants when it is not possible to include all of the potential people who could inform the evaluation. This involves a systematic form of selection designed to avoid bias. The evaluation team may deliberately, or (more commonly) inadvertently, select participants who are likely to have the views and opinions they are hoping to see, for example they may select nurses they consider to have a favourable view of clinical supervision and its implementation.

If the evaluation team is able to administer the survey or questionnaire(s) to all nurses who have been involved in the implementation of clinical supervision (and the control group if applicable) then there is no need for sampling. While it is preferable to include the total population, often insufficient time and financial resources mean that this is not possible.

Probability or random sampling is typically regarded as the most rigorous approach to sampling for statistical research. This is because every person in the population has a chance of being selected, avoiding the possibility of researcher bias. For example, if simple random sampling is used, the evaluation team would assign a number to every nurse who could potentially be a participant in the study. Random numbers are then computer generated and obtained from a random number table. The nurses represented by the numbers generated through this process become the sample.

Power analysis

The primary purpose of evaluating clinical supervision is to determine whether or not this intervention has resulted in positive outcomes for nursing and health care within an organisation. Often the primary focus is of local interest, meaning that if the evaluation team feels clinical supervision is effective according to the measures used, this may be sufficient. However, if the team is interested in considering the potential value of clinical supervision more broadly within nursing or the health care system, then it is important to be confident that the findings are likely to be reliable and valid.

Power analysis and sample size estimation enable the evaluation team to determine the sample size required to make accurate and reliable statistical judgements. It also assists in determining the size of any observed effects (i.e. small, medium or large). By conducting power analysis and sample size estimation, the evaluation team can determine the number of participants they need to ensure that the sample is sufficiently large to draw meaningful conclusions.

Further reading

If you require further information about power analyses, see Cohen (1992).

Cost-effectiveness

In order to convince managers and administrators that clinical supervision is a wise investment, it is likely that you will be expected to demonstrate cost-effectiveness. This is particularly important if clinical supervision is to be sustained in the longer term.

Demonstrating the cost-effectiveness of any health care initiative is neither simple nor straightforward, and clinical supervision is no exception. At the very least it would be advantageous to demonstrate that the introduction of clinical supervision is cost neutral. The successful implementation of clinical supervision involves the investment of considerable financial resources to provide education and training, and the release of both supervisees and supervisors from clinical duties. In Chapter 3 the cost of time release alone was estimated at $A10 000 per month for a rural mental health service.

Reflective exercise

Estimate the cost of providing clinical supervision for nurses on the unit or team where you work according to the minimum recommendation of 1 hour per nurse per month.
You will need to:

- estimate the average hourly rate per nurse (human resources may be able to provide this information)
- multiply by the number of nurses per unit/team
- multiply by two (to include both supervisors and supervisees).

This calculation gives the approximate cost. It is likely to be conservative as it is quite likely that supervisors will be more senior and therefore paid at a higher rate to the supervisees.

Whether or not the figure surprises you, it is likely to equate to a significant investment of resources. While you may appreciate that the benefits of clinical supervision go beyond those that can be demonstrated as a financial saving, the financial managers of the organisation will probably need further convincing. Improved patient care and increased productivity, for example, are difficult to prove and even more difficult to assign a dollar value to.

Since we know that clinical supervision costs money, demonstrating cost-effectiveness means that financial savings of at least equal value must be demonstrated. Potential areas for demonstrating cost-effectiveness include:

- reduced absence from work due to illness or stress
- decrease in staff turnover
- a reduction in the number of critical incidents such as medication errors, aggressive incidences.

The advantage of this form of evaluation is that the data should be collected routinely and are not difficult to access. Unfortunately, we are subject to the same difficulties in interpreting results as we find with surveys and questionnaires. For example, if a reduction in absence due to illness or stress is evident, can we be confident that clinical supervision is responsible? These rates vary for many reasons, as do the figures for staff turnover.

Critical incident rates have their own challenges; it is not unusual to notice an increase following the introduction of an initiative such as clinical supervision. While this may give the impression that errors, accidents or other untoward events have increased, and possibly that clinical supervision has negative outcomes, it is generally more an issue of reporting than of incidence. For example, through receiving clinical supervision nurses who have previously considered verbal or physical violence as part of the job may come to see it as a challenge that needs to be overcome, with reporting as the first stage of this process.

Multimethod approach

Interpreting the results of research and evaluation involving human participants must always be treated with a degree of caution. People are inherently complex; their attitudes, opinions and behaviours do not occur in isolation, and therefore isolating the precise cause of any observable changes is difficult, perhaps even impossible. For example, a reduction in critical incidents and sick and stress leave, and improved retention rates may be claimed as a positive consequence of introducing clinical supervision. In reality, however, there may be another cause that has not been identified or controlled for, such as a change in management, improved working conditions, or perhaps an unusual trend that is relatively short term, with apparent changes that would tend to even out over time.

While no particular method of data collection will enable full confidence that the results reflect the introduction of clinical supervision, the more extensive the data collection is, the more likely it is that consistency in results has been influenced by this initiative. Ideally, an evaluation would use a combination of in-depth interviews with multiple stakeholders, surveys and methods to determine cost-effectiveness. However, economic reality suggests that sufficient funding would probably not be available to support this. Given these constraints the evaluation team will need to strike a balance between the type of information they would like to collect and what they can afford to collect.

Conclusion

If clinical supervision is to be successfully implemented and sustained a systematic evaluation must be an inherent part of the process. There are a range of methods that can be used as part of an evaluation strategy.

Qualitative and quantitative approaches both have a lot to offer as well as some significant limitations. A mixed method approach using multiple collection techniques will be more likely to produce results that, if consistent, could be indicative of the impact of clinical supervision. Economic constraints mean that not all possible data collection techniques are likely to be utilised.

References

Boynton, P.M. & Greenhalgh, T. (2004) Hands-on guide to questionnaire research: Selecting, designing, and developing your questionnaire. *British Medical Journal*, 328, 1312–1315.

Cohen, J. (1992) A power primer. *Psychological Bulletin*, 112(1), 155–159.

Finch, H. & Lewis, J. (2004) Focus groups. In: Ritchie, J. & Lewis, J. (eds). *Qualitative Research Practice: A Guide for Social Science Students and Researchers*. London: Sage Publications, pp 170–198.

Happell, B. (2007) Focus groups in nursing research: An appropriate method or the latest fad? *Nurse Researcher*, 12(2), 19–24.

Kevern, J. & Webb, C. (2001) Focus groups as a tool for critical social research in nurse education. *Nurse Education Today*, 21(4), 323–333.

Legard, R., Keegan, J. & Ward, K. (2004) In-depth interviews. In: Ritchie, J. & Lewis, J. (eds). *Qualitative Research Practice: A Guide for Social Science Students and Researchers*. London: Sage Publications, pp 138–169.

Maslach, C. & Jackson, S. (1986) *The Maslach Burnout Inventory*. Palo Alto, CA: Consulting Psychologists Press.

McHugh, G. & Thoms, G. (2001) Patient satisfaction with chronic pain management. *Nursing Standard*, 15(51), 33–38.

Posavac, E.J. & Carey, R.G. (2007) *Program Evaluation: Methods and Case Studies*. (7th edn). Upper Saddle River, NJ: Pearson Prentice Hall.

Reed, J. (2005) Using action research in nursing practice with older people: Democratizing knowledge. *Journal of Clinical Nursing*, 14(5), 594–600.

Weiss, D.I., Dawis, R.V., England, G.W. & Lofquist, L.H. (1967) *Manual for the Minnesota Satisfaction Questionnaire, Work Adjustment Project, Industrial Relations Center*. Minnesota: University of Minnesota.

Winstanley, J. (2000) Manchester Clinical Supervision Scale. *Nursing Standard*, 14(19), 31–32.

Index